THE TRUTH
ABOUT CANCER

To Inge

with every good wish

from

[signature]

25ᵗ October 1989

THE TRUTH ABOUT CANCER

A PERSONAL GUIDE
TO CAUSES AND TREATMENT

Dr Jan de Winter

BLANDFORD PRESS

POOLE · NEW YORK · SYDNEY

First published in the UK 1986 by Blandford Press
Link House, West Street, Poole, Dorset, BH15 1LL

Distributed in Australia by
Capricorn Link (Australia) Pty Ltd
PO Box 665, Lane Cove, NSW 2066

British Library Cataloguing in Publication Data

De Winter, Jan
    The truth about cancer.
    1. Cancer
    I. Title
    616.99′4   RC261

ISBN 0 7137 17793

Typeset by Lovell Baines Ltd, Hollington Farm, Woolton Hill,
Newbury, Berkshire.

Printed in Great Britain by Biddles Ltd, Guildford

For
Oma, Edith,
Michi and Daniele

CONTENTS

Annual deaths per 100 million Americans aged under 65.

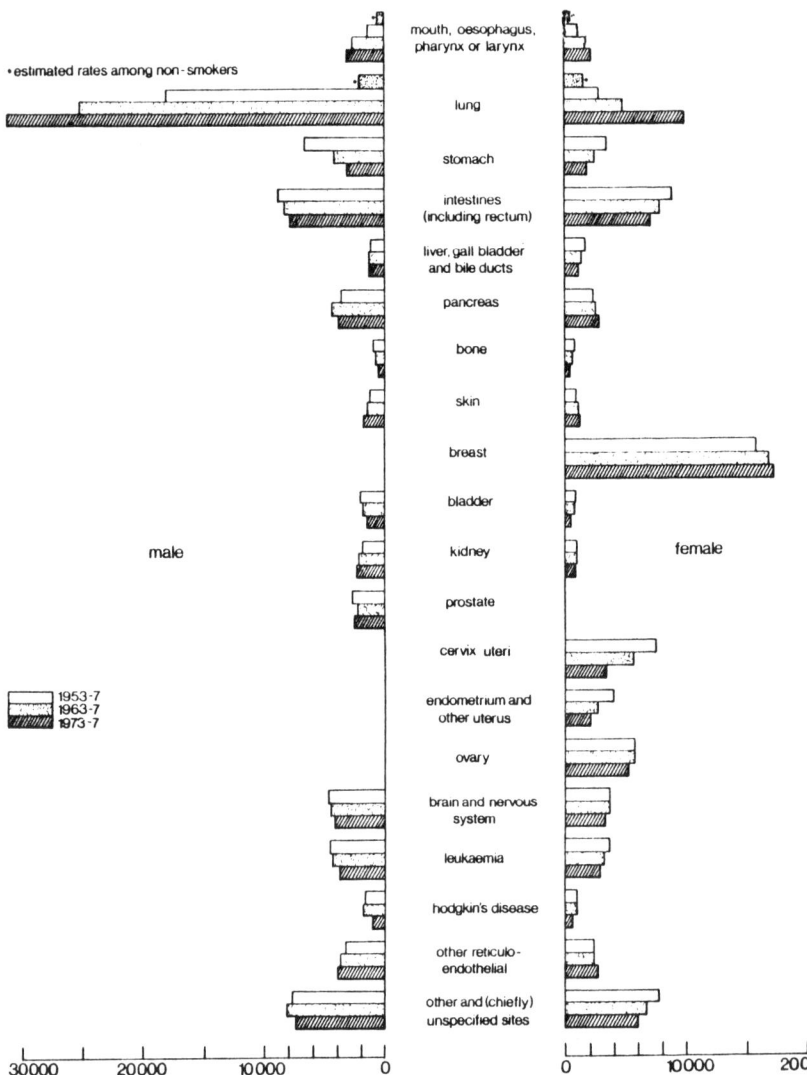

* estimated rates among non-smokers

male

female

1953-7
1963-7
1973-7

mouth, oesophagus, pharynx or larynx
lung
stomach
intestines (including rectum)
liver, gall bladder and bile ducts
pancreas
bone
skin
breast
bladder
kidney
prostate
cervix uteri
endometrium and other uterus
ovary
brain and nervous system
leukaemia
hodgkin's disease
other reticulo-endothelial
other and (chiefly) unspecified sites

30000 20000 10000 0   0 10000 200

The cited rates are per 100 million people under 65; since there are at present about 100 million Americans of each sex aged under 65, the cited rates are similar to the actual numbers of middle-aged Americans that die of these diseases each year. (After *Cancer; Risks and Prevention* by MP Vessey and Muir Gray, Oxford University Press 1985)

INTRODUCTION: LOOKING AHEAD WITH HINDSIGHT

As long as we allow the word cancer automatically to imply a hopelessly progressive and generally fatal disease, allied to unrelievable suffering, no real progress in its control can be expected. This defeatist attitude, by anticipating the outcome, virtually paralyses the forces in us which protect our good health and help us in our recovery from ill-health.

This misunderstanding of the word cancer can create such nervousness in otherwise sensible people that they come to believe that contracting the disease is the will of God or some kind of retribution for past misdeeds – a threatening condition that singles out its victims one-by-one. Reactions may differ wildly. At one extreme, people may decide to burn the candle at both ends, 'having a jolly good time while the sun still shines'. At the other, they may live all the time under a dark cloud of fear that can actually increase the likelihood of developing the disease.

Because cancer currently affects one person in three in the Western world, most families have a first-hand knowledge of the suffering the disease can inflict both on the victims and their relatives. Having witnessed the ravages cancer can cause to the once-healthy body of a relative, a dear friend or neighbour, the horrified onlooker can be left with a lasting impression of gruesome suffering. It is this terror-inspiring memory which gives cancer such a frightening reputation.

These nightmare fantasies, when coupled with fear, can sometimes create a totally unnecessary reaction against the poor, unsuspecting cancer victims, who frequently and quite wrongly, are looked upon by relatives as contaminated carriers of a contagious disease. As a direct result they may find themselves shunned by both their own relatives and their friends; they may even be allotted separate cutlery, crockery and linen and told to use a toilet and bathroom which is not to be used by anyone else. This marks them as outcasts and makes them feel unwanted, which indeed they mostly are.

Unlike patients with heart disease, which is equally lethal but not

9

shameful, cancer patients have to lie (and be lied to) because the speaking of the word is still so repugnant. By the attitudes which surround it, cancer can threaten one's family relationship, one's love life, one's chances of promotion and even one's job. So patients with the disease frequently have no alternative but to become secretive. This negative attitude to cancer has a generally depressing effect on people and this sense of despondency is deepened by newspaper and television reports of heroic but unsuccessful battles of individual cancer patients, who eventually succumb because of the odds against them.

The unfortunate effect of these chilling messages often extends to the relationship between cancer patients and those relatives, friends or professional advisers who genuinely try to help them. Not knowing how to relate to the cancer patient, and in the mistaken belief that it is catching, friends often prefer to stay away altogether. Many people also do not wish to be reminded of death. Most relatives feel awkward and inadequate in the presence of a cancer patient and this attitude only further contributes to the patient's feeling of helplessness and foreboding.

Even doctors can become somewhat inept in the presence of cancer patients. They frequently avoid answering the patient's questions and try to comfort them with half-truths in the face of what they regard as inevitable death. Not unnaturally, the doctor's attitude is sensed by the patient. The message is clear: the patient will not survive.

This climate of doom surrounding everything relating to cancer has very grave consequences as regards early treatment. For instance, when a person discovers a lump, he or she, for reasons quoted above, will often be too frightened to reveal its existence until it can be concealed no longer. By then it is generally too late. A few actual clinical histories will illustrate this point:

1. A woman aged 58, the wife of a voluntary car driver bringing patients to a radiotherapy department, was too frightened to go to her doctor and eventually did not even allow her friends into her house, because she had been concealing, for over three years, a large ulcerating tumour of the right breast, which had invaded the chest wall so deeply that onc could see the aorta pulsating at the bottom of the ulcer crater. It was only when the husband could stand the offensive odour no longer that he consulted a doctor, but at this late stage nothing could be done.

2. A woman aged 36 concealed a large ulcerating tumour of the left breast for two years by wearing large dressings on the wound and by

padding the left cup of her brassiere. She slept in a separate bedroom from her husband and was too frightened to speak to anyone about her tumour, including her own doctor. Eventually her sister surprised her in her bedroom while changing the dressing and she was successfully treated.

3. A woman who had a tumour had attended a faith healer for 18 months. By the time she was seen by a physician it had invaded the whole of the left chest wall and hung 13 inches down to the pelvis. The patient was convinced that since it was not painful it would go away. Furthermore she trusted the 'healer' to take out the poison. Had she spoken without delay to her doctor, whom she had not seen for years, the outcome would probably have been different. As it was, no treatment was possible because of the extent of the tumour.

4. A pipe-smoking man aged 52, successful in business, the father of four teenage children, with a very happy family-life and heavy financial responsibilities, concealed first a lump in the tongue and subsequently a secondary gland at the side of the neck, until profuse bleeding from the tongue could no longer be concealed from his family. According to the patient, this haemorrhage occurred at least two and a half years after he first noticed a swelling on his tongue, situated exactly where the tip of his pipe-mouthpiece pressed on the tongue. At first, he thought that he only imagined the swelling, but when it grew larger, he realised its ghastly significance, having previously been told by a doctor-friend about the association of pipe-smoking and mouth-cancer.

Because of his heavy financial commitments in respect of school fees, a large mortgage, three cars, expensive holidays and a luxurious life-style, he felt compelled to stay in his job and not to run the risk of a reduction in income while away receiving treatment or having an operation.

By the time he attended hospital he was in great pain, the lump in the tongue had ulcerated and there was a plum-sized swelling of the gland in the neck below the angle of the jaw. He received a six weeks' course of radiotherapy and subsequently an only partially successful attempt at surgical removal of the neck-gland was made.

He survived for barely one year, the last stages being greatly complicated by constant pain, requiring regular morphia medication.

There is only a very brief period before tongue-cancer becomes incurable and that period occurs right at the start, well before the appearance of an enlarged lymphgland. Once lymphgland involvement has occurred, curative treatment is rarely possible.

5. A 28-year-old female patient who had been bleeding for over twelve months was too frightened to visit her doctor. She also felt that she could not talk to him because he was too busy in surgery hours; she wished there was a medical person somewhere to whom she could go and talk at leisure without feeling she was being a nuisance. She was brought to the radiotherapy department on a stretcher, via the emergency department, having fainted in the street due to serious blood-loss. No treatment was possible because of the advancement of a cervical growth.

Of course, it stands to reason that the sooner a course of treatment for an established cancer is started, the greater will be the chance of success. What is less obvious, yet equally important, is the individual's mental approach to the whole problem of cancer from the time he or she first discovers the name of the disease.

There are still far too many people who believe that each person is earmarked by destiny for or against developing cancer. This is not so. However, what is certain is that being full of apprehension and concern about one's own future acts against remaining cancer-free. To be permanently anxious or worried is to invite trouble through suppression of the body's own immunological defence mechanism. This system, which protects us against ill-health, works best when our mind is care-free, when it is clear of negative emotions like stress, fear, resentment or despondency.

The mind therefore plays a vital role in helping the body to subdue cancer. It might help to imagine the ever-present cancer threat living in each of us as an evil crab. The crab has a two-pronged attack, firstly by its powerful claws and secondly by its deadly poison. The strength of our healthy body can keep the crab's claws in check, and our positive attitude of mind can stop the flow of poison. The body *and* the mind must join forces; either one or the other alone is not able to cope with the crab's double attack.

It is well to remember in this context that the quality of health we enjoy is not something that others can give us; we have to find it for ourselves.

Medical history teaches us that the major scourges in the past were overcome not by some stupendous medical discovery but rather by remarkably unglamorous, self-imposed changes in our own life-style.

For instance, the cholera epidemic of the last century, and other equally lethal infections, were eliminated by the very ordinary means of improved public health measures and higher standards of personal hygiene.

This century's scourge is cancer and again it is likely to be overcome by similarly low-key, subtle changes in our behaviour pattern, particularly in the field of nutrition.

The major obstacle to progress in this century, as last, is the lack of public enlightenment and the lukewarm response on the part of the community to recommended changes. The current, almost total public apathy is illustrated by a recent US Government poll which shows that 49 per cent of the US population continue to be unaware of what to do to prevent cancer, and that another 46 per cent believe that nothing can be done. Yet it can be shown that even very minor changes in our eating and living habits could reduce the deaths from cancer by at least 25 per cent by the year 2000.

So far, the cure for cancer has eluded us and such a discovery will remain beyond our reach until we know much more about cell growth. This will take decades, if not another century.

In the absence of a cure for cancer we have to rely on prevention. It has been shown that this can be achieved through close attention to eating and living habits, provided there is sufficient motivation and willpower. In short, to succeed we must *want* to do it. There are many people who, while enjoying good health, will see no need to change their way of life. They will say that they are happy the way they are and so far nothing bad has happened, so why change? This argument is short-sighted. The habits damaging to our good health, which can eventually bring about cancer, will only produce deterioration in our tissues if carried on over many years. At first these changes are unnoticeable, and more important, reversible; but if the bad habits persist they build up and the destruction does eventually become irreversible. Therefore, it is absolutely vital to alter one's faulty life-style before this point is reached.

To understand this better we may compare it with the sport of boxing. What counts as regards lasting brain damage is not the number of knock-outs a fighter experiences but the number of blows to the head. All of these blows will cause *some* structural damage to the brain and each blow will increase the damage. In other words, the damage will be cumulative.

This has been suspected for many years, but it has remained undetectable until the recent development of a revolutionary X-ray scanning procedure. Called *computerised axial tomography*, it can examine the brain in thin 'salami-slices', section by section. As a result of this examination, the damage has now become detectable long before it shows itself in outward symptoms, such as slurred speech, or uncoordinated movements and other serious neurological disorders.

Similarly, the small, early changes eventually leading to cancer currently continue to remain undetectable at a time when they are still reversible, that is, while the ultimate change to a malignant growth has not yet taken place and the disease is still avoidable.

There are many who, on principle, object to any imposed change of life-style as an interference with individual liberty. They will point out that it is perfectly legal to damage oneself with alcohol, nicotine and other permitted drugs, so why not with food? After all, committing suicide, whether by instant violence or by the more drawn-out means of neglect and gluttony, is not illegal. If people wish to damage their health, they will say, it is no one's business but their own.

But once the disease has struck, this utterly stupid attitude soon changes and is replaced by a feeling of guilt and remorse. The situation resembles the British public's attitude to seat-belts before the recent introduction of legislation. For many years there had been an excellent case for motorists to wear seat-belts. Yet it took two decades and thousands of casualties to overcome public opposition to legislation, but within a few months of its introduction, the immense benefits in the saving of life and limb, and also of money, have become clearly apparent. The results in cancer prevention will be neither as quick nor quite as obvious. But the case for introducing such measures to avoid cancer is equally important. The first step is one of public relations, because only when people have become fully aware of the damage that they are doing to themselves will there be a better chance for a change of heart. This change must come before any telling change in life-style.

This book is a serious health warning to encourage readers to make the necessary adjustments to their own life-style, before any damage becomes irreversible. Once we have learned what to do, all that will be required is a small daily extra effort of will-power and self-discipline. However, to keep this up we need to have a full understanding of what cancer is all about. Therefore, the second aim of this book is to provide knowledge about the disease. Origin, causes, nature, types, treatment, side-effects, success, failure and prevention will all be discussed. Then readers can decide for themselves whether or not to follow the more disciplined lifestyle outlined in Chapter 13.

1·THE NATURE OF CANCER

Body cells, which are the building bricks that make up the 'house' of the human body, reproduce themselves by cell division in a remarkably controlled fashion.

Some cells reproduce faster than others. For instance, the cells of the skin, or the cells that make up the blood or those that line the walls of our intestines display the fastest rate of division in an effort to replace those which have been worn out or damaged. This cell reproduction is done according to a masterplan in which cell death matches cell production. We are still not sure how this is achieved.

Sometimes it happens that some families of cells increase their numbers at the expense of their neighbours. It is when, in so doing, they invade their neighbour's territory, that they are to be regarded as cancerous cells.

Cancer is assumed to arise in a single cell, in fact in a small area of a single cell called the *gene*, consisting of a protein called DNA which carries the *genetic code* of each cell. Once this cell starts dividing abnormally, all the cells coming from it will continue to reproduce in an uncontrollable fashion. This change in a gene which produces such abnormal cell division is called a *mutation* and the agent that brings about such a change is called an *initiator*. In order to mature into a cancerous growth the presence of another factor is required; this is called a *promoter*.

The nature of both an initiator and a promoter is not known with any certainty. It can either be a factor in the environment, a chemical substance, a persistent damaging personal habit, or possibly even a virus. Although the nature of the mutagenic (cancer-causing) factors is unclear, it is certain that the presence of both an initiating and a promoting agent is necessary for activation of the cancerous process. In the absence of either, malignant growth does not occur.

The fact that cancer is more frequent in older people tends to support

15

the idea that there are a number of controlling genes in the cell which prevent it from forming an ever-expanding family of cells. It is thought that only when these controlling genes have been destroyed one after another by separate mutations over many years, will cancer arise in one of the normal cells.

It is also thought that the probability of this mutation is likely to increase the more it has been exposed to oddities of lifestyle or bad habits. Therefore the older we are the greater the likelihood of a mutation in a controlling gene.

Once this loss of genetic control has taken place, the rate of multiplication of new cells will no longer match the rate of loss of old cells; it will exceed it and this results in tumour formation.

It is frequently assumed that the tumour grows because its constituent cells divide faster than its normally-controlled healthy counterparts. The answer is that more of them remain in the dividing pool of cells where they continue replicating. In normal circumstances they would have differentiated and ceased to reproduce.

One of the controlling mechanisms is known; it is called *contact inhibition*, and its job is to stop a cell from dividing as soon as it comes into contact with its neighbouring cell. This contact inhibition appears to operate no longer for cancer cells.

A well known example of this type of control can be seen in the skin. Here cell division usually takes place only in the basal layer of the cells which separates the top layer, called *epidermis*, from the underlying layer of loose cells, called *dermis*.

Cells are seen to divide only in the basal layer and once outside it they are discarded or they die. Cancer cells, on the other hand, do not seem to receive or obey controlling signals and they continue to divide even outside the basal layer or when in contact with each other.

This wide range of uncontrolled behaviour is shown by cancers that arise in the sheets of epithelial cells found in the lungs, respiratory tracts and intestines or forming glands such as breast, pancreas, thyroid, prostate, ovary or testis.

Let us take the breast as an example. It is the strong interaction between epithelial cells and the supporting tissue, called *stroma*, which determines the behaviour of epithelial cells in the breast. When breast cancer develops, different divisions of a single mammary gland invade each other's territory and reproduce to invade the surrounding tissues.

Clinically two groups of cancers are recognised, one called *carcinomas*, because they arise in epithelial cells and the other *sarcomas* which develop in tissue supporting bone cells, blood vessels, fibrous tissues and muscle.

There is a mixed group of cancers arising in the lymphatic system and bone marrow which comprise Hodgkin's Disease, lymphosarcoma and leukaemia respectively. Over 90 per cent of human cancers are carcinomas and less than 10 per cent are sarcomas and leukaemias. It is of interest that in children (and in animals) leukaemias and sarcomas are the most common.

There are over 200 distinct varieties of cancer; yet one half of all deaths from cancer are due to only three forms. These are cancer of the lung, cancer of the large bowel and cancer of the breast. Mercifully all three are at the head of the list of avoidable cancers.

Each cell is made up of a basic protein called DNA. This protein can be regarded as the genetic blueprint for subsequent generations of cells, which all will resemble the original cell in every single aspect. This is made possible by a neat arrangement on cell reproduction, whereby the DNA of the mother cell ingeniously arranges itself into two parallel chains and on cell division each one of these chains becomes incorporated in the daughter cell, where the genetic blueprint will be reproduced and this pattern is followed down the line from one generation of cells to the next. Because each single detail of a mother cell re-appears in the daughter cell, any fault that may be present in the mother cell, will necessarily be passed on and emerge also in the daughter cell. Such faults or changes are called mutations and when they occur in certain parts of the DNA chain they are thought to be responsible for the creation of cancer cells.

There are two general types of cells, namely those of which all organs are made up, the body cells or somatic cells, and those of the germline, which make up the sperm or the ovum. On fertilisation the fertilised cell will be made up of half of the chain from the sperm and half from the ovum. Any defect that is present in both the sperm and ovum cells will re-appear in the cell resulting from the fusion of the two chains on fertilisation.

If such defect is present only in either the sperm or the ovum, it may be compensated by the absence of the defect in the other half and thus may disappear. Such a defect is called recessive. If, on the other hand, the defect is too powerful to be compensated, it will re-appear and such a defect or mutation is called dominant and it will be passed to the offspring.

Somatic cells with defects can only harm the host, whereas a dominant defect in a germline cell will harm the foetus.

There are many agents capable of producing these changes. The simplest is the effect caused by ultraviolet light which causes adjacent parts of a gene to become tied together. Since the ultraviolet light of the sun does not penetrate deeply it can only affect genes situated in the cells of the skin and eyes. By contrast, X-rays (which are penetrating) can produce mutations in any part of the body.

CHEMICALS

Another group of harmful agents are chemicals. For instance, there is the substance called *benzpyrene*, which becomes linked to one part of a gene and is a known cause of cancer.

Benzpyrene is a member of an important group of compounds called *polycyclic hydrocarbons*, substances purified from tar, which are made up of hydrogen and carbon. These substances are very widespread in nature; they are produced, for instance, in fat that has been used repeatedly for frying food, or in any process involving heating organic matter either by burning it quickly, as in burnt toast or a barbecue, or warming it slowly over millions of years, as in the warm oil and coal deposits.

In their natural form these compounds do not react chemically with DNA. After entering the body they are detoxified in a succession of steps. It is then that they become unstable and act as powerful mutagens because they can readily interact with DNA.

The body is well protected against the effect of these harmful mutagens. In the skin or the intestine this protection is provided by the mechanism of the constant shedding of the surface layers of cells. This rapid loss of epithelial cells from the surface (which is compensated by a high rate of cell division in the superficial layers) is the body's inbuilt protective device against any harmfully active environmental compound. Those compounds that are instantly reactive are least dangerous because they will be shed with the superficial layers. It is the more stable ones, like benzpyrene, which do most harm. These will be absorbed by the body unchanged and only become reactive as they break down.

Certain enzymes which are produced in the body in response to substances which in themselves are not carcinogenic, are available to be used in the breakdown of chemical carcinogens as well. Such substances are called *inducers* and they are used in the testing of various chemical compounds for carcinogenicity. It is no longer necessary to use live animals for these tests: a new and totally revolutionary technique employs simple bacteria on *Agar* plates. It is only necessary to add a suitable activating enzyme (inducer) which will make the bacteria susceptible to mutation. Such tests, which used to take at least a year when animals were used, now take one day only and are quite inexpensive. The speed ensures routine testing by all major chemical manufacturers of all their new compounds before they are put on the market. Testing has become as rapid as it is reliable and it is possible to predict the carcinogenicity of new substances with a high degree of accuracy. Had these tests been available at the time of the discovery of tobacco, it would have been possible to foresee its risks in the causation of lung cancer, as it is such a powerful carcinogen.

THE SLOW GROWTH OF CANCER

Another characteristic of some cancers is their long induction time. This means the interval between the start of operation of a carcinogenic stimulus and the final appearance of the tumour which tends to be decades rather than years. For example: people have to smoke between 10–20 years before lung cancer develops; leukaemia usually develops seven years after accidental exposure to X-rays; vaginal cancer in teenage girls occurs some 15 years after birth, as a result of previous stimulation, due to high doses of oestrogen(s) given to their mothers during pregnancy and which passed through the womb to the unborn foetus.

It would seem that particularly rapidly dividing cells, under pressure of prolonged excessive hormonal stimulation, can, after many years of such regular provocation, make mistakes in genetic control which will eventually lead to mutation. This change appears to depend on the balance between gene repair and speed of reproduction. Cells with little time to spare for repair between each cell division are of greater mutagenic sensitivity, and this may be one reason why cancer occurs mostly among especially rapidly dividing cell populations.

However we still do not know why it is that some forms of cancer grow faster than others, why some are more invasive than others or why some tend to metastasise or spread, while others do not, even when they arise in areas next to each other. For example, cancer of the lip rarely metastasises, whereas cancer of the tongue tends to spread to lymph nodes at an early stage. Similarly, cancer of the hard palate has a better forecast than cancer of the soft palate, because it does not involve regional lymph nodes so readily.

Cancer of the body of the uterus mostly remains there, but cancer of the cervix tends to spread much more readily.

There are three types of skin cancer of which only one, the melanoma, which arises in the skin's pigment cells (called melanocytes), is dangerous on account of its tendency to distant blood-borne spread. The other two types, because they rarely metastasise, are extremely curable. They are the rodent ulcer, which arises from the basal layer of the skin, and the squamous carcinoma, which arises from the more superficial squamous skin cells.

2·WHAT WE SHOULD KNOW ABOUT CANCER

When cancer strikes, the shocked patient's senses may be too numbed by the implications of her (or his) affliction to ask some obvious questions about her future, in particular about the chances of survival, the type, duration, side-effects and success-rate of treatment and how much of this to tell to relatives or friends.

Even the most experienced and compassionate cancer specialist, who has the patient's peace of mind very much at heart, may find it difficult to give a clear explanation, because so much will depend on the presence or absence of metastases. This is the one overriding factor that will determine the success or failure of the treatment.

TREATMENT BY SURGERY

If surgery is the recommended treatment, then removal of the growth usually means removal of the organ in which it arises, sometimes together with removal of the regional lymph nodes as well. Post-operative recovery is quick, rarely extending beyond ten days, by which time all stitches in the skin will have been removed from the suture and the wound should have healed soundly.

Surgery can only be performed when the tumour is actually operable. Sometimes this cannot be determined in advance by physical examination and in these circumstances the surgeon must actually open up the patient in the operating theatre and have a look under sterile conditions before a decision to operate on the cancer can be made. However, the implications of surgery should be discussed openly before the patient agrees to the operation, and alternative types of treatment should be explained.

It is easy to see that, for surgery to be successful, all the tumour must be removed. If it is so large as to occupy most of an organ, provided that it is compatible with survival, that organ is best removed together with the tumour. If it is very small and the organ can be preserved, only the tumour is removed with a good margin of surrounding healthy tissue.

TREATMENT BY RADIOTHERAPY

Radiotherapy uses tissue-penetrating rays to destroy the tumour *in situ*. Naturally some damage is inflicted on the tissues and organs in the path of the rays and this produces both a local response and a more generalised reaction. The local reaction of the skin consists of tissue-inflammation and irritation, sometimes resulting in the shedding of the covering layers, and exposing of a tender, raw, bleeding surface. The speed of recovery for the bruised tissues depends on the amount of exposure to the rays, and on the sensitivity of the affected organ. The brain, skin and some of the pelvic organs, such as the uterus and the bladder, are quite resistant to radiation. On the other hand, the eyes, lungs, liver, kidneys and rectum are less so, and sometimes suffer permanent damage.

In addition to the direct local tissue reaction, there is the body's general reaction which makes the patient feel unwell, a condition sometimes described as 'radiation sickness'. The severity of this reaction mainly depends on three factors. First and foremost is the radiation dose received each day and the total dose of a full course of treatment. This is important, since the radiation effect is a cumulative one and the unpleasantness of the reaction increases with time, to become most pronounced towards the end of treatment and for a week or two after its completion.

The severity of the reaction will also greatly depend on the area being irradiated, because the more tissue included in the beam of penetrating rays, the worse the reaction will be. The dose that is absorbed in a given volume of tissue is called the *integral dose*. Only a limited integral dose is compatible with survival. Finally, the actual site of irradiation is of vital importance as regards reaction. For instance, treatment of the head or the extremities does not produce half as much in the way of radiation sickness as is experienced when the trunk and, in particular, the abdomen are being irradiated.

Radiation sickness consists of a feeling of tiredness, nausea, lack of appetite and sometimes vomiting and depression. During irradiation of the abdomen, diarrhoea sometimes develops.

The severity of these symptoms (which can be relieved by drugs) depends very much on the patient's attitude to treatment and his or her morale. Patients who are despondent and resentful at having to have

22

treatment usually suffer far more from radiation side-effects than those who are cheerful, optimistic and confident.

TREATMENT BY DRUGS

The third recognised form of treatment for cancer is by means of drugs, and here again the side-effects are frequently the limiting factor as regards the length and intensity of treatment. The reaction on *chemotherapy* (as drug treatment is sometimes called) resembles that experienced on radiotherapy, and that is why the effect of drugs is sometimes referred to as being *radio-mimetic*. Additionally, there is the morale-sapping drug effect of total, though usually temporary loss of hair. It is possible, as with radiotherapy, to relieve the unpleasantness of the side-effects by prescribing certain medicines and vitamins. Again, as with radiotherapy, the severity of side-effects varies from patient to patient and is lessened by the patient's positive attitude to treatment.

UNORTHODOX TREATMENT

Some patients with cancer seek the help of medically unqualified practitioners, in preference to having orthodox treatment. All these patients will come to regret this fatal error because, in so doing, they will forfeit the only chance that they may have of a cure.

There is one elementary guide-line to be rigidly adhered to by all cancer patients. Never try unproven methods first; if they are to be tried, they should be left until after orthodox treatment has been completed. In this way the chances of a cure will not be sacrificed.

SUCCESSFUL TREATMENT

As has already been stated, although it is essential to start treatment as soon as possible, a permanent cure for cancer depends on there not being any new satellite growths at distant parts of the body. Surgical removal of a growth with a view to a cure can be considered only in the rare case where the disease 'permits' this by remaining localised to its site of origin.

Similarly, the other two available treatment methods (radiotherapy and chemotherapy) can be used with success only when the tumour is composed of cells which happen to be more sensitive to damage by radiation or by drugs than the most sensitive normal cells of the body.

The result is that the malignant ones can be destroyed before permanent damage is inflicted on the normal ones.

This unsatisfactory state of affairs will continue to thwart our best efforts until we have learned to make the most of the body's own resources in controlling the disease.

WARNING SIGNS

In the average person's mind cancer is seen as a mute disease which creeps up with the stealth of a thief on the unsuspecting victim and which makes its appearance totally unexpectedly, mostly when it is already too late.

This impression is not altogether correct. It is true that in its earliest stage cancer is usually silent. However, as soon as it has reached barely visible proportions, it betrays its presence by a number of warning signs. If these signs are not to be missed, they must be learned, kept in mind and looked out for, without apprehension or hysteria, but nevertheless constantly.

There are about seven general symptoms which although not exclusively indicative of cancer, may sometimes represent early warning signs of the disease and should therefore be assumed to be due to cancer, until proved otherwise.

1. The most important sign is unusual bleeding or discharge from any part of the body but particularly from the nose, mouth, ears, or the urinary, vaginal and back passages. Such bleeding will be discussed in greater detail when describing cancer at the various sites.
2. A thickening or lump in the breast, testes, tongue or elsewhere must be suspected to be due to cancer, until disproved.
3. Similarly, an ulcer or sore, which is a defect in the skin or other tissues is very suspicious of malignant disease, particularly when healing is delayed, and must be further investigated.
4. A change in bowel habits – either constipation or diarrhoea – lasting for more than a week, as well as a change in bladder habits such as frequency, urgency or difficulty in passing water, requires search for the cause. These signs may be due to a malignant change in the intestines and in the gynaecological or urinary tracts respectively.
5. A stubborn huskiness of voice, a persistent hoarseness, or a particularly obstinate cough lasting for more than three weeks, are very suspicious and the cause must be investigated.
6. Difficulty in swallowing, as well as persistent indigestion and lack

of appetite are signs of possibly serious abnormalities in the gullet or stomach; since its causes are relatively easy to determine, medical advice should be sought at an early date.

7. Finally, a pre-existing birthmark or mole which shows signs of activity by increasing in size or deepening in pigment or by starting to bleed is suspicious of malignant change, and must be investigated at once.

Contrary to popular belief, the symptom of pain rarely figures among the early signs of cancer. This is mainly because the haphazardly dividing cancer cell which is of inferior quality, not being masterminded by the body's genetic code, matures without receiving a nerve supply which would enable it to communicate with the brain. Only when the tumour's bulk compresses or invades neighbouring structures which *do* possess a nerve supply, is a painful stimulus relayed and pain registered by the patient, something that occurs in the later stages of cancer as a rule.

The only painful early sign, which may indicate the presence of a tumour, is headache; this is because of the rigid structure of the skull, which tightly envelopes the brain. Therefore, any increase in volume also increases the intracranial pressure to give headaches, particularly in the morning on waking. If associated with nausea, vomiting or blurring of vision, instant advice must be sought.

General tiredness, sudden loss of weight and extreme weakness are popularly believed to be the most typical signs of cancer. They are in fact late, frequently pre-terminal signs of cancer and indicate the general spread of the disease due to the breakdown of the patient's immunological defence mechanism. This is followed by the collapse of most of our normal physiological functions, leading to an irreversible decline.

PROGNOSIS

One of the most important questions that can ever be asked by a patient suffering from a potentially lethal disease such as cancer, concerns the success of treatment. In this respect, however much the doctor may wish to put the patient and relatives at ease, it is not possible to state confidently that a cure is guaranteed, because each patient responds individually and there is the agonising uncertainty regarding the presence of distant spread which may so far not have revealed itself.

Certain forms of cancer carry a favourable prognosis. They include in particular the four rarer forms, affecting mainly the young adult, namely: Hodgkin's Disease, testicular tumours, choriocarcinoma and acute lymphoblastic leukaemia in children. Among what are called solid tumours, the ones carrying a good prognosis are epithelial cancer of the skin, cancer of the lip, cancer of the larynx and cancer of the cervix.

It is important to be as truthful as possible in circumstances where the whole truth is not known. It helps greatly if the doctor takes the patient totally into his confidence. Only when there is total understanding between patient and doctor and when he enjoys the full support of his relatives can the patient's morale be kept high.

One of the questions frequently asked of a doctor is to what extent a patient will be able to resume a career after treatment. On this point the answer can usually be very reassuring, provided the disease was in an early stage and is of a type which is known to respond to treatment. What should be uppermost in everyone's mind is the realisation that the fact that the patient contracted active cancer is a sign that there was something in his career and living habits, which taxed the body's immunological defence mechanism beyond endurance. If one accepts this to be true, then when discussing the patient's return to work, one should ensure that the factors which sapped the patient's resistance to cancer should be removed from his everyday life. This is vital because the chances for the patient's long-term well-being are intimately bound up with his resolve to take full responsibility for his own body, both physically and spiritually.

3·THE MOST COMMON CANCER SITES

CANCER OF THE BLADDER

The bladder is a muscular sac that stores and empties urine which has been carried down the two tubes (called ureters) from the kidneys. The urine is emptied by the bladder through another tube (called the urethra). In women this is very short and runs in front of the vagina; in males it is much longer, passing through the prostate and along the under-surface of the penis. One of the main contributory causes of bladder cancer is smoking, since some of the breakdown products of tobacco are excreted in the urine.

SYMPTOMS

The prime symptom of bladder cancer is blood in the urine (*haematuria*). It mostly appears quite suddenly and without pain. Depending on the amount of blood, the urine may vary from a smoky- or rusty-shade to deep red in colour but the amount of blood is not related to the stage of advancement of the disease. Sometimes haematuria may be due to a stone or to bladder-infection. It is important to realise that the urine may often remain clear for weeks or months after the initial bleeding, but with bladder cancer it will reappear sooner or later. If blood clots form they may block the urethral opening and cause painful bladder-muscle spasms.

DIAGNOSIS

The diagnosis is established by means of a *cystoscope*, a slender rod fitted with a lens and a light that works in a similar way to a periscope. The cystoscope is inserted through the urethra into the bladder where tissue from suspicious-looking areas can be removed for examination under a microscope.

TREATMENT

The treatment of established bladder cancer is tailored to the individual needs of the patient; the most important points being the type, location and advancement of the disease, as well as the patient's general condition. A solitary mushroom-type tumour (called papillary) can be removed by a wire loop and the base *cauterised*; this procedure can be carried out through a cystoscope. Such patients have to have regular cystoscopies, as further papillary tumours may appear in other parts of the bladder. When several such tumours are found they are usually treated by surgical removal of the affected section.

When the tumour has spread over most of the inner surface or when it has grown right through the bladder wall, the entire bladder may require removal by surgery (*cystectomy*). A number of methods have been developed to provide a substitute store for the urine. The most common one is for the surgeon to shape a new bladder from a segment of small intestine. Both ureters are attached at one end and the other end is brought out through the wall of the abdomen near the navel where it forms an opening, called a *stoma*. A flat bag attached to the skin with a special type of glue is placed over the stoma and serves to collect the urine.

At first many patients are apprehensive, and embarrassed at having to wear a bag. It does take some getting used to, but within a few months, except when having to empty the bag, most patients are scarcely aware of it. The bag is not visible under casual clothing and does not prevent a person from returning to work, taking part in sports or even swimming.

The alternative treatment for advanced bladder cancer is radiotherapy, usually a daily treatment for about six weeks. Although the radiation is carefully beamed (by pin-pointing the target with the help of the CAT scanner) to include the bladder only, a side-effect in the form of troublesome diarrhoea is almost inevitable as the rectum lies immediately behind the bladder. The radiation-induced inflammation of the bladder-lining also adds to the patient's discomfort when urinating. As at other sites, results of the treatment of bladder cancer, whether by cystectomy or radiotherapy, depend on the advancement of the disease. Chemotherapy is not used in the treatment of bladder cancer as, so far, no sufficiently effective drugs have been discovered.

CANCER OF THE BONE

Most of the skeleton is composed of bone which forms a rigid framework bearing the weight of the body. A malignant tumour which develops in the skeleton is known as bone cancer.

There are two main classes of cancer: the carcinomas which develop in the lining and covering tissue of organs, and the sarcomas which develop in the connective and supportive tissues of the body. Bone cancers are usually sarcomas. Most common childhood bone tumours are *osteogenic sarcomas* which appear usually in the bones around the knee. *Ewing's sarcoma*, also a children's cancer, usually affects the mid shaft of bones. These childhood cancers will be discussed in the next chapter.

Bone cancer in adults is usually secondary to a primary tumour elsewhere in the body, which has spread to the site via the bloodstream. On rare occasions cancer can extend to the bone from adjacent tissues. Secondary bone cancers are much more common than cancer which starts in the bone and they usually originate in the breast, lung, thyroid and kidneys. The areas usually affected by the secondary growth are the spine, the ribs, the pelvis, the skull and the upper thighs.

SYMPTOMS

Unlike cancer at other sites, pain is the symptom most noticeable in bone cancer probably because of the rigidity of bony tissues which cannot expand when pressed on by an invading tumour. The pain from bone cancer is usually worse at night. The most frequent sites are the thigh, knee, pelvis, upper arm, ribs and vertebrae. Swelling or fever may accompany the ache and if it affects the lower limbs there may be repeated unexplained stumbling.

Primary bone cancer mostly affects children and early symptoms are usually dismissed as either a sprain or growing pains. In older patients, who have already learned to live with aches and pains, cancer of the bone is frequently discovered only when a tumour-weakened bone fractures.

TREATMENT

Treatment of bone cancer can involve all three interdependent approaches of cancer-control surgery, radiotherapy and drugs. In the case of osteogenic carcinoma, amputation of the limb at least eight centimetres above the point where X-rays show cancerous cells is usually recommended. Present day amputees usually return to normal ability very quickly, being fitted with a light-weight *prosthesis* or artificial limb, in many cases held on by suction.

Both chemotherapy and radiotherapy may be used along with surgery. Some patients with osteogenetic sarcomas may be treated with high doses of special anti-cancer drugs which cause hair loss, nausea and vomiting, as well as inflammation of the lining of the mouth. The course of drug treatment may take anything up to two years. After treatment medical examinations are carried out regularly to monitor for a recurrence of the disease.

BRAIN CANCER

The brain is enclosed within the hard casing of the skull. With one exception, cancer that begins in the brain does not metastasise to other parts of the body, yet the brain is a common site for a metastasis from elsewhere.

SYMPTOMS

The most common first symptom of a brain tumour is persistent headache; this is caused by the increasing pressure of the growing cancer on normal brain tissue. Headaches may be associated by increasing irritability or unusual sleepiness. The more rapidly the tumour grows the more disturbing the symptoms it causes. These include nausea, vomiting, loss of hearing, taste, balance, sight, speech or control of movement. Sudden *epileptiform* seizures and temporary loss of consciousness occur in about one-third of brain cancer cases.

DIAGNOSIS

The diagnosis of a brain tumour starts with the examination of the optic nerve which connects the retina of the eye with the brain. An ophthal-moscope is used to look at the retina. A tumour compressing the nerve results in swelling of the nerve-ending in the retina; this is called *papilloedema*. The clinical examination is completed by examination of muscle function, reflexes and ability to feel pinpricks.

The greatest recent advance in brain tumour diagnosis is the CAT scan, which allows detailed examination of the brain in thin cross-sectional slices. The brain's electrical activity can be recorded by a method called electro-encephalography (or EEG). Electrodes are attached to the scalp and electrical readings are recorded by the machine. (Both the CAT scan and the EEG are totally painless and the patient feels nothing at all.) If the picture of the CAT scan is not clear some tissue may be removed for examination to confirm the diagnosis.

Sometimes the arteries supplying blood to the brain are outlined by a dye and an X-ray is taken; this is called *angiography*. The purpose is to detect a change in the usual pattern of these arteries caused by their displacement as the tumour grows. This examination is carried out under anaesthetic and is not painful.

TREATMENT

Brain tumours can be treated by surgery, radiotherapy, anti-cancer drugs and a combination of these methods. Surgery is the oldest method and a neurosurgeon can sometimes remove a cancer that is encapsulated in a membrane and so cure the condition. If the whole of the tumour cannot be removed, part of it will be cut away to relieve the pressure that the growing tumour is causing within the skull and with it the unpleasant persistent headache. Radiotherapy is used mainly to shrink the tumour and reduce pressure inside the skull.

Chemotherapy is hampered by the blood-brain barrier that prevents anti-cancer drugs (with the exception of a new group called *nitrosoureas* which are especially effective in reaching the brain) from getting through the walls of the brain arteries. Only temporary relief has so far been achieved by chemotherapy.

CANCER OF THE BREAST

Breast cancer, with 40,000 cases in Britain and 90,000 in America every year is the most common form of female cancer. It will affect one woman in thirteen and at present 13,000 women a year die of breast cancer in the UK alone.

The type of woman most prone to be attacked by the disease is probably overweight and childless, with a history of menstrual problems stretching over 40 or more years. The frequent onset of breast cancer at the time of the menopause is probably caused by the hormonal imbalance associated with the 'change of life'.

Another important factor is the consumption of too much dairy produce (whole milk, butter, cream and cheese) which makes the body produce too much of the enzyme lactase. This enzyme is known to be involved in the development of breast cancer. Having a close relative with breast cancer also increases the risk of contracting the disease but this is not as important as being childless. In other words, having a child is very protective and this explains why breast cancer is so common in nuns.

The commonest breast problem, namely lumpy breasts, may or may not indicate a higher risk; no one is quite sure yet on this point. It is therefore advisable to be watchful and carry out frequent self-examinations and when in doubt, to see a specialist and even ask for an X-ray. On the other hand, what we know for sure is that a woman who has had breast cancer in one breast is six times as likely to get it in the other breast; of course, this risk can be reduced by a suitable change in eating and living habits. A patient who continues living in an identical fashion before and after successful treatment for breast cancer is really encouraging the development of a second tumour.

SYMPTOMS

When trying to pin-point the early signs of breast cancer a woman should look out, first and foremost, for an unusual, firm, round lump (tumour) in the soft tissue of either breast. Sometimes only puckering, dimpling or scaliness of the skin can be detected. Ulceration of the skin is a more advanced sign, as is retraction of the nipple. Stains (pink or clear) on underclothes or brassiere, suggest a discharging nipple which must be investigated at once. Any change in the size or shape of the breasts can be quite serious and requires urgent attention.

SELF-EXAMINATION

Since one woman in 13 is likely to develop breast cancer, every woman should pay special attention to the breasts by practising self-examination at the same time each month, shortly after the end of her period when the breasts are least active. This applies equally to women who have completed the menopause. It is a simple procedure and consists of feeling the breasts with two finger tips as well as visual inspection.

First, in a standing position, one hand should be raised in the air and using two fingers of the other hand, the opposite breast should be gently explored feeling for any unusual thickening or lumps under the skin. This should be repeated on the other side. Secondly, standing in front of a mirror both breasts should be checked for any signs of puckering, dimpling or of a scaly skin. Leaning forward the breast should be checked for any abnormalities in shape. The nipples should be inspected for evidence of any discharge. Lastly, the fingertip check described above should be repeated, this time lying flat on the back with one arm behind the head. A small pillow should be placed under the shoulder blade of the side to be examined, to flatten out the breast on the chest wall for easier checking.

DIAGNOSIS

In women known to be at risk from breast cancer it may be vital to detect the disease even before a lump can be felt. Several techniques are available for this: the two most common methods use X-rays, either on film (*mammography*) or on paper (*xeroradiography*). Another method, *thermography*, measures the heat from the breast; an increase in temperature in one breast may indicate an abnormal condition, such as cancer. However, these methods can only suggest the possibility of cancer. As at other sites, the final diagnosis is always made from a piece of suspect tissue.

If a lump is present a simple procedure is to suck some cells from it through a needle (this is called *aspiration biopsy*). If only fluid is present and the lump collapses when punctured, a diagnosis of a simple cyst is made.

TREATMENT

Once cancer is definitely established, treatment will have to be discussed with the patient, because some women may not be able to come to terms with a breast amputation (*mastectomy*). This used to be the standard operation for breast cancer until a few years ago and women were obliged to accept the loss of a breast since no alternative method appeared to offer similar results. Fortunately this is no longer so. Provided the tumour is smallish in comparison with the remaining breast, and provided it is situated conveniently at the outside of the breast, any patient may now demand to have the lump removed (*lumpectomy*).

The treatment results are similar but many surgeons still prefer to remove the whole breast, instead of just taking out the lump. A six-week course of post-operative radiotherapy following lumpectomy is usually needed, particularly when enlarged lymph nodes in the armpit are present or suspected. Sometimes these are removed together with the breast lump.

About ten per cent of woman who undergo mastectomy have lasting serious anxiety, depression or even sexual problems afterwards that justify reconstructing the breast. Not all women are able to have this operation and it is not advised in patients who have had a mastectomy for an advanced growth. Reconstructive surgery is not usually carried out for at least a year after treatment which included radiotherapy. However, there are some surgeons who favour reconstruction at the time of operation.

Reconstruction is an attempt to produce a convincing mound that will match as nearly as possible the volume, position, mobility and shape of the opposite breast; this does not include reconstruction of the nipple.

The actual surgical procedure after a simple mastectomy consists of inserting a silicone-gel prosthesis between the chest wall and the overlying pectoral muscle. At body temperature the silicone has a consistency of normal breast tissue.

Sometimes, women request reconstruction of the nipple. This can be done either with the help of a graft from the opposite nipple or, alternatively, an adhesive nipple can be used to give the necessary 'button' beneath the blouse or brassiere.

Taking stock of treatment results in breast cancer reveals the same story: the more extensive the disease, the less chance for cure. In the final analysis, the final result will, as always, hinge on the distant spread of the disease (metastases) and no one knows or is likely to find out in the foreseeable future how metastases come about. Since they are as frequent after a mastectomy as after a lumpectomy, unnecessary mutilation, which can cause such a blow to a patient's feeling of femininity, should be avoided at all costs. In this respect, the patient's wishes should be paramount.

When the tumour has progressed beyond the earliest stages and has spread outside the breast and armpit lymph nodes, only relief treatment is possible. Radiotherapy, hormone therapy and chemotherapy will then all have a role to play, either alone or in combination.

In breast tumours which are hormone-dependent, treatment by hormones is preferred and can be effective for many months. This form of therapy is usually free from unpleasant side-effects and is therefore always worth trying. Before hormone therapy of younger women is started, the ovaries are generally removed to deny cancer cells their source of growth-stimulating hormones. After the menopause removal of other hormone-producing glands, such as the adrenal glands at the top of the kidneys, or the pituitary gland at the base of the brain, may be considered. However, because of the severity of the surgery and its limited success, these major operations have now gone out of fashion.

Breast cancer metastases favour the bony skeleton, particularly the spine, the pelvis and the thigh bones. The sometimes excruciating pain associated with bone metastases is readily relieved by local radiotherapy. A bonus is that such treatment also helps to prevent a fracture at the site of the metastasis due to tumour-erosion of the bone, because the soft bone, *decalcified* as a result of invasion, is able to *recalcify* and become hard again.

The role of chemotherapy in breast cancer is still being considered and several useful drugs are being studied. A new development is the use of long-term oral drug therapy, either in healthy volunteers, or after surgery. The drug is administered in small doses without side-effects. This is an attempt to prevent the disease altogether, or to improve the indifferent results of treatment in most of the early cases of breast cancer.

Little progress has been made in breast cancer cure-rate over the past 40 years and therefore prevention, by means of a diet low in all types of fat, but in particular milk-fat, should form part of health education of every young woman.

Since breast cancer is the most frequent form of malignant disease in women and since early breast cancer, when treated promptly, offers the best chance of a cure, monthly breast self-examination should be practised by every woman. The nature of any breast lump should be discovered by examination of cells or a piece of tissue under the microscope.

CANCER OF THE COLON AND RECTUM

The large bowel consists of the colon and the rectum through which solid and semi-solid waste is passed. The colon is about 150 cm (5 ft) long and the rectum occupies about the last 15 cm (6 in) of it.

SYMPTOMS

There are several early signs of colonic or rectal cancer but the main one is blood in the stools which can be bright red, dark red or black in colour. Other symptoms are a change in bowel habits such as diarrhoea or constipation and occasionally abdominal discomfort or pain.

DIAGNOSIS

A tumour in the rectum is within the reach of a doctor's examining finger and will therefore be found by rectal examination. To confirm this the tumour can be viewed by means of a *proctosigmoidoscope* through which it is possible to see the lower twelve inches of the bowel where many tumours of the large bowel occur. A sample of tissue (*biopsy*) which is taken for examination under a microscope will confirm the diagnosis. This can also be confirmed by introducing a contrast medium (*barium enema*) into the bowel and taking a series of X-rays which may reveal an obstruction. In another test, a search is made for hidden blood in the stools; this is analysed in the laboratory. More recently, the *fibre-optic colonscope*, a highly flexible tube no thicker than a finger which can be moved through the curves and around the bends of the colon, has made the examination of the entire bowel possible.

TREATMENT
Cancer of the colon sometimes starts with a small cherry-like polyp suspended on the intestinal wall. This is easily removed through the colonoscope and if proved malignant more extensive surgery will be required. Sometimes it will be necessary to perform a *colostomy*, which means an opening of the bowel through the skin surface of the abdomen to allow body waste to be removed. The colostomy may be either a temporary or a permanent one. The temporary one is usually carried out to permit the bowel to rest during the time required for healing. If a large part of the colon including the rectum has to be removed the colostomy will be a permanent one and the patient will need to wear a colostomy bag. At first, this is repugnant to many patients but eventually, with patience, most people become accustomed to managing their lives without being too upset by having to dispose of their soiled plastic colostomy bags.

Sometimes radiotherapy is used instead of surgery and at other times it can be used before an operation to help shrink the tumour. This makes the operation much safer. Occasionally a course of X-ray treatment is recommended as a follow-up to surgery, especially when the rectum has been removed. Finally, in advanced cases when surgery is not possible, palliative radiotherapy is an effective means of relieving pain due to the growth.

Chemotherapy will have to await the discovery of new drugs before it can be used more extensively in the treatment of advanced bowel cancer.

HODGKIN'S DISEASE
Hodgkin's Disease is a form of cancer affecting the body's lymph nodes

which form part of the general circulatory system. The main role of this lymphatic system is its ability to fight infection on our behalf.

SYMPTOMS

Hodgkin's Disease usually begins as a painless swelling in one or more lymph nodes, often the neck, although the armpits and the groin are also favourite sites for the first appearance of enlarged lymph glands.

These lymph glands manufacture *lymphocytes*, which are white blood cells concerned in the fight against the spread of infection. In Hodgkin's Disease these white cells grow rapidly in a variety of abnormal forms; this growth takes place at the expense of the normal lymphocytes and leaves the body with too few to fight infection. The patient with Hodgkin's Disease is therefore prone to contracting infectious illnesses such as flu or the common cold far more readily than the average healthy person.

It is assumed that Hodgkin's Disease starts in one lymph node and spreads from there to affect other lymph-node areas. As it progresses the patient becomes weaker, anaemic and less able to combat infection.

Any enlarged lymph node, particularly if situated in the neck, armpits or groin, remaining swollen for more than three weeks, should be investigated, as it may well be due to early Hodgkin's Disease. Other illnesses can also start with lymph node enlargement such as glandular fever. It is therefore most important to establish the actual cause of such lymph node enlargement at an early date so that appropriate treatment can be started promptly. All other symptoms of Hodgkin's Disease are late ones and include fever, tiredness, loss of weight, itching and night sweats, the latter two signs being of particularly serious significance.

DIAGNOSIS

The diagnosis is usually made as a result of special X-rays, blood tests and biopsy.

Once the nature of the disease has been confirmed, the extent of lymph node enlargement throughout the body must be found out. This is called *staging* and its accuracy determines the degree of long-term success of treatment.

TREATMENT

The type of treatment is chosen according to the stage of the disease.

Usually the patient is submitted to a CAT scan which reveals previously invisible structures such as enlarged lymph nodes in the abdomen. It is particularly important to check the presence of glands along the spine in what is called the *retro-peritoneal space*. If this is uncertain the patient is subjected to a *laparotomy*, a diagnostic operation during which an incision is made in the skin over the abdomen; this enables the surgeon to examine the whole abdominal cavity. A smaller operation of the same kind is called *peritoneoscopy*, during which a slender fibre-optic instrument is inserted through a slit in the skin of the abdomen to examine the internal organs and take tissue samples of suspect areas.

Once staging is completed the crucial decision about treatment can be made. The disease is classified into four stages according to its extent. When enlarged lymph nodes are confined to one area it is classified as stage one. When two adjacent areas are involved it is called stage two. Stage three has been reached when the disease affects the lymph node regions above and below the diaphragm. Once Hodgkin's Disease is found to have spread to other organs such as lung, bone, liver or kidney – that is stage four. Each of these stages is sub-divided into groups A and B, according to whether or not the patient experiences such general symptoms as weight loss, fever or night sweats.

Stages one and two are usually treated by radiotherapy alone. Stages three and four are usually treated by chemotherapy but a combination of both treatments can be used, depending on the response of the disease.

Hodgkin's Disease is eminently curable in the early stages and up to 77 per cent of stage one cases have remained permanently cured. As in all cases of malignant disease, follow-up examinations at an early date, when the disease is still confined and treatable, are of vital importance to detect any renewed flare up.

Patients with Hodgkin's Disease may remain immunologically deficient for many years after treatment and may therefore be subject to more frequent infections. To remain permanently free of the disease they will have to take special care of both their physical and mental well-being and try not to run unnecessary risks by over-straining their physical or spiritual resources.

CANCER OF THE KIDNEY

Cancer of the kidney, also called *hypernephroma* or *renal cell carcinoma* is more common in men than in women. It is difficult to diagnose early and as a result less than 30 per cent of patients can expect to be cured by a combination of surgery and radiotherapy.

SYMPTOMS

About two-thirds of patients exhibit symptoms of blood in the urine and/or low, one-sided backache. The other third of patients experience more general symptoms such as fatigue, fever or loss of weight. Another late symptom is a lump or mass that can be felt in the area of the kidney.

DIAGNOSIS

When kidney cancer is suspected, several tests can be carried out to confirm it. The most important one is the *intravenous pyelogram*. For this, iodine-containing dye (which will be concentrated and excreted by the kidneys) is injected intravenously. This will help to show up not only a mass in the kidney, but also how the kidneys are functioning. An ultra-sound examination, using sound waves, helps to distinguish between a cystic (and probably benign) mass and a solid, malignant one. Sometimes an *arteriogram* is performed to discover the blood-supply to the kidney. This involves the injection of a dye into a tube that is passed up an artery in the leg right up into the region of the kidney. By revealing the blood-supply of the cancer, the surgeon gains important information about how to approach the cancer at operation.

Before the best type of treatment can be worked out, one must ensure that the disease has not spread to distant parts of the body. For this, a chest X-ray as well as a bone and liver scan are necessary.

TREATMENT

If the cancer is found to be localised to the kidney, a *nephrectomy* (removal of the kidney) together with a removal of the nearby lymph nodes is recommended. Post-operative radiotherapy to the kidney-bed is administered as a routine in more advanced cases.

In patients with metastatic kidney disease, treatment is still disappointing because both drugs and hormones remain ineffective at present.

CANCER OF THE LARYNX

SYMPTOMS

One of the commonest symptoms of laryngeal cancer is huskiness or hoarseness and therefore any long-term change in one's voice should be investigated. Other symptoms are a change in the voice-pitch, the feeling of a lump in the throat, coughing, difficulty in breathing or swallowing and sometimes even ear-ache.

DIAGNOSIS

The diagnosis is readily made by using a laryngeal mirror similar to that used by a dentist. At the same time, the presence of enlarged lymph nodes in the neck is looked for by the doctor. The malignant nature of the growth is confirmed by removing a sample of tissue for a biopsy.

TREATMENT

The treatment for a localised laryngeal growth is radiation therapy for which a six weeks' course is usually given. During the latter half of the course, the patient will probably lose his or her voice, have a very sore throat and will find it difficult to swallow. But the voice returns and swallowing becomes easier within three to six weeks of completion of treatment. The results of radiation therapy for early carcinoma of the larynx are excellent.

For more advanced growth, surgery is sometimes used. There are two types of operation: the more limited one is called *partial laryngectomy* where only part of the larynx is removed, usually leaving a normal or only slightly hoarse voice. If it is necessary to remove all of the larynx, a *total laryngectomy* is performed and the upper air passage (*trachea*) is stitched to an opening in the skin (*tracheostomy*) so that air can pass through this to enter the lung. After operation the patient usually breathes through this opening rather than through the nose and mouth. Sometimes it is necessary also to remove enlarged lymph nodes in the neck called *neck dissection*. It is to these tissues and not to distant parts of the body that cancer of the larynx will spread.

After total laryngectomy the patient will have to learn to speak again by a technique known as *oesophageal speech*, which is produced by expelling swallowed air from the oesophagus. A great deal of training is necessary to acquire an oesophageal voice which will produce good-quality speech and the method is best learned from a qualified speech-therapist. There are mechanical devices, such as an artificial larynx, for those patients who are unable to learn the method. A mechanical larynx is a device that converts air motion into sound. It is held up to the hole in the neck that is left when the larynx is removed. Speech with this device is easy to understand but it has no normal inflections.

Although results of radiation treatment of early laryngeal cancer, as already stated, are excellent, long-term cures after total laryngectomy for advanced growth are less good. All patients must attend for follow-up examinations regularly, at first every three months and then at longer intervals.

ADULT LEUKAEMIA
Leukaemia can occur at any age and affects children and adults in different ways. In the adult there are two main forms of leukaemia depending on which of the two kinds of white cells the cancer affects, the *lymphocytes* or the *leucocytes*. There is also a chronic and an acute form of each.

SYMPTOMS
Chronic *lymphocytic leukaemia* develops slowly, mainly in elderly people. Symptoms are so mild that the diagnosis is usually a chance finding, discovered during a routine blood test. When symptoms do occur they are both vague and generalised in nature – such as fatigue, lack of energy, fever, loss of appetite and weight, night sweats or anaemia. These can be associated with enlarged lymph nodes in the neck or groin and an enlarged spleen, which can be felt under the left ribs.

The signs of chronic *myeloid leukaemia* which arises in the other white cells, the *leucocytes*, are similar to those of chronic lymphatic leukaemia. They are usually more pronounced, but as a rule the disease is again discovered accidentally.

The symptoms of the two acute forms progress far more rapidly; there is bone pain, paleness, a tendency to bleed or bruise and lymph node or spleen enlargement.

DIAGNOSIS
The diagnosis of all four forms is made on a blood test which usually shows *blast cells* (immature cells), as well as a low red and white blood cell count. An *aspiration biopsy* of the bone marrow (withdrawal of blood cells through a needle from the breastbone or pelvic bone) will be necessary to confirm the type of leukaemia and its degree of malignancy. It also is used to monitor the progress of treatment.

TREATMENT

The acute forms of leukaemia are treated by *combination chemotherapy*, using a number of drugs simultaneously. This achieves destruction of cancer cells without permanent damage to the normal blood constituents. Unfortunately, the advances made in the successful treatment of children's acute *lymphoblastic leukaemia* have so far not been emulated in the adult leukaemias.

When malignant cells accumulate in the brain (where due to the unique properties of the blood vessels they might be safe from the drugs), radiotherapy to the brain is used to destroy them. If the disease recurs, the original abnormalities reappear and then it is common for a tendency for bruising and bleeding to develop. Chronic lymphocytic leukaemia has the better prognosis and such patients may be left untreated without risk for many years.

Side-effects from the drugs used may introduce a number of complicating problems. If the reproduction of platelets in the bone marrow has been damaged by the drugs, a platelet transfusion may occasionally be necessary to prevent bleeding. Sometimes platelets are withdrawn from a recovering patient and these are then frozen. If they are required after a relapse, they are re-injected into the patient.

Similarly, in case of a low white count, and associated proneness to infection, a transfusion of white cells can be given with beneficial effect. It is difficult, however, to obtain these cells in adequate amounts from normal blood donations. To control this increased liability to infection patients are now isolated in special germ-free rooms.

CANCER OF THE LUNG

Like most forms of cancer, lung cancer is also an expression of uncontrolled growth. It usually arises in smokers as a result of chronic irritation of the lining of the air tubes (bronchi) by the tar, which is transported into the lungs in cigarette smoke on inhalation.

SYMPTOMS

The early diagnosis of lung cancer is influenced by the fact that nearly all lung cancer patients have been cigarette smokers and have had a bad cough or bronchitis for years. A cough is also the major symptom of cancer. Although some smokers believe to have noticed a change in the quality of their cough from a loose one to a more hacking-kind of dry cough a few weeks or months before their lung cancer was discovered, this is by no means a constant or reliable finding. What is a warning sign of cancer, though rarely an early one, is the presence of blood in the spittle causing a streakiness of the saliva with a rusty or even bright-red colour.

Chest pains can occur in the form of a dull ache which may or may not be related to coughing. Wheezing or hoarseness are also late symptoms as are repeated episodes of infection such as pneumonia or bouts of flu. Generalised symptoms of advanced lung cancer include, as in other cancers, fatigue and loss of appetite and weight.

DIAGNOSIS

Since there are no unmistakable early signs of lung cancer, it is essential that all smokers have a chest X-ray at least once a year. Because of the presence of air in the lungs, even a small tumour shows up relatively early.

Once lung cancer is suspected on X-ray, the bronchi are examined with an instrument called the *fibre-optic bronchoscope*. This is a thin flexible tube which can be threaded deep down into the larger branches of the bronchi and which enables the examining specialist to see the inside of the tubes by means of a viewer like a tiny television screen. During the *bronchoscopy* a bit of the suspicious tissue is usually removed for examination under a microscope.

Another test available is examination of the spittle for malignant cells. This is an adaption of the popular Pap test which has proved to be of such value in the early diagnosis of cancer of the cervix.

TREATMENT

The choice of treatment for lung cancer depends on the advancement of the growth. All three routine forms of treatment can be employed. The first, surgery, is rarely applicable because only rarely is the tumour sufficiently localised to make possible complete removal of the growth which may sometimes include removal of the nearby lymph nodes too. In more advanced cases a whole lobe or an entire lung may have to be removed. However, the results are poor.

When surgery is not possible, radiation therapy in the form of super-voltage x-rays are used to destroy as much of the cancer as possible, with minimal damage to surrounding normal tissue. Radiation therapy is mainly used to improve the quality of life by relieving distressing symptoms.

The third form of treatment, sometimes used in conjunction with surgery or radiotherapy, is chemotherapy which uses drugs to kill

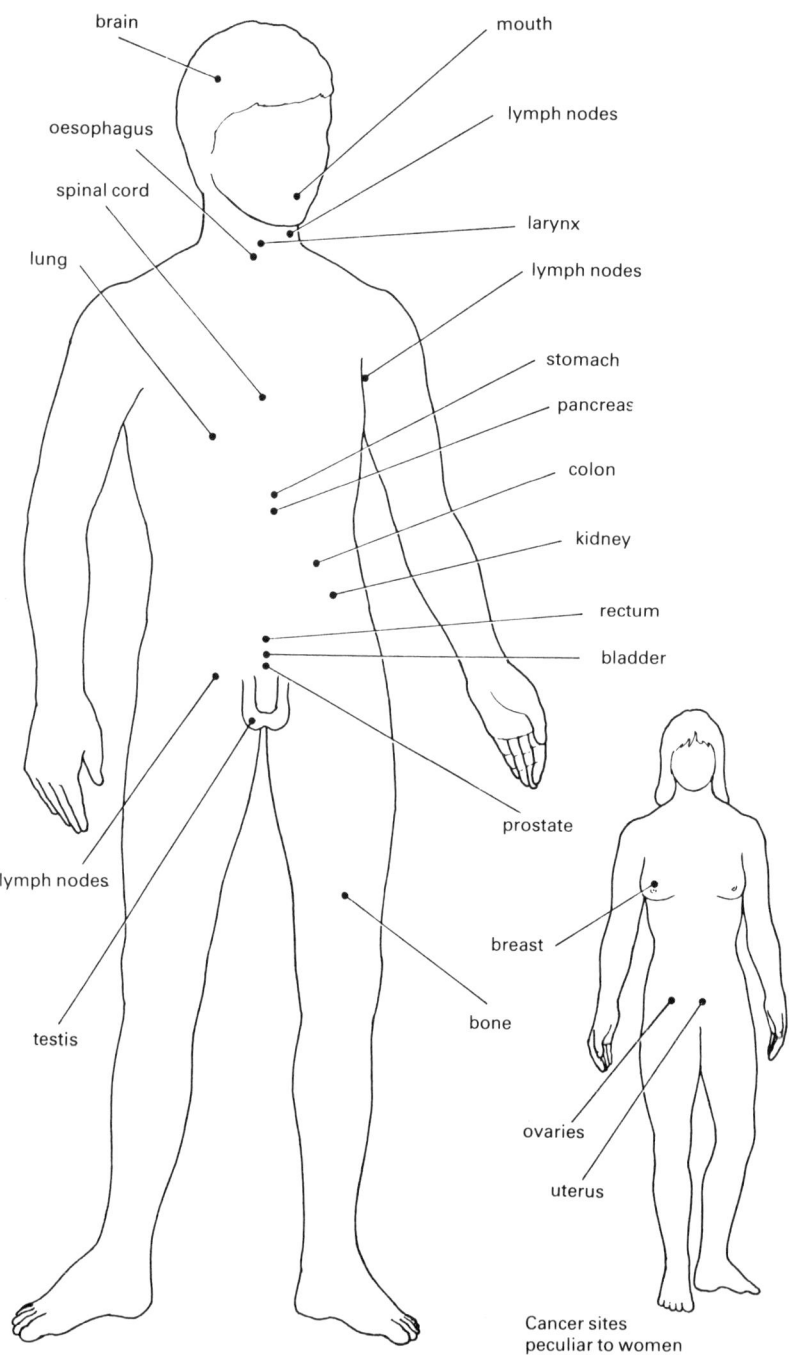

brain

mouth

oesophagus

lymph nodes

spinal cord

larynx

lung

lymph nodes

stomach

pancreas

colon

kidney

rectum

bladder

prostate

lymph nodes

breast

testis

bone

ovaries

uterus

Cancer sites
peculiar to women

44

cancer cells. How much is given and how often depends on the type of cancer to be treated, the type of anti-cancer drug prescribed, how well the drug is tolerated and how long it takes to respond to it. It is not unusual that drug treatment has to be stopped due to its unpleasant side-effects.

Treatment results in lung cancer are disappointing because in the lungs the tumour can advance silently, beyond a stage where it can either be totally cut away or completely removed by radiation. Regular check-ups are vital because the disease has a habit of recurring, sometimes locally, sometimes at a distant site, most frequently in the brain which seems to be a place favoured by lung metastases.

With such a poor treatment record it is incomprehensible, now that we know the close causal relationship between smoking and lung cancer, that many more people do not decide to stop smoking.

CANCER OF THE MOUTH

SYMPTOMS
Cancer of the mouth, also sometimes referred to as cancer of the oral cavity, includes cancer of the lips, tongue, soft and hard palate and floor of the mouth. All of these sites are easily visible and readily accessible, therefore any abnormal areas which persist more than two weeks must be reported. Such abnormalities include a swelling or a lump, a rough patch, brown or black spots, a sore that does not heal, or continuous bleeding. The diagnosis is made by a biopsy.

A *leucoplakia*, which is a thickened piece of epithelium, appears as a white patch in the membranes covering the tongue, lip or floor of the mouth. It is not malignant but may develop into cancer. Anyone with a leucoplakia must stop smoking or the chances of developing cancer in the mouth will be even greater. Any such persistent white patch must be biopsied and checked regularly for the possible development of cancer.

TREATMENT
Surgery is used in many cases to remove the tumour; often the nearby lymph nodes are removed at the same time. Radiotherapy is the alternative treatment, given either by external radiation or, as in the case of tongue cancer, implanting radioactive sources into the growth (called *interstitial radiation therapy*).

Radiotherapy is sometimes used before an operation to shrink a large tumour to a more operable size. At times post-operative radiotherapy is employed for cancer cells the surgeon could not reach at operation. The side-effects of radiotherapy are difficulty in chewing and swallowing, a reduction of the amount of saliva in the mouth and a loss of sense of smell and taste. Such symptoms are only temporary and their duration depends on the size of area treated and X-ray dose administered. Complete recovery usually takes between four and six months.

Chemotherapy is rarely used in cancer of the oral cavity. The best results of treatment are obtained when the tumour is small and there are no nearby enlarged lymph nodes.

MULTIPLE MYELOMA

Multiple myeloma is a cancer that arises in one type of white cells, the plasma cells in the bone marrow, which is the soft sponge-like material in the centre of the bone. The function of plasma cells, which form part of the body's immune system, is to fight infection by producing antibodies. When plasma cells start growing in an abnormal manner and form malignant tumours, they stop producing antibodies and the body loses resistance to infection. As a result the patient becomes prone to colds, coughs, flu, pneumonia and other infections.

SYMPTOMS

The first sign of multiple myeloma is pain in the bone, usually backache. Later the pain may shift to the ribs, neck or pelvic areas.

By crowding out the red cells and platelets in the bone marrow, the patient can become anaemic and tired, as well as having bleeding gums and frequent nose bleeds. Other late symptoms are bone fractures and painful pressure on the spinal cord.

DIAGNOSIS

The diagnosis is made from blood and urine tests, which show the presence of abnormal proteins. Examination of the bone marrow can detect increased numbers of cancerous plasma cells. The specimen of tissue is obtained by means of a bone marrow biopsy, during which a special needle is inserted into the breast bone or pelvic bone and a small amount of tissue is taken for examination in the laboratory. X-rays of the skeleton show up the areas of bone invaded by the malignant plasma cells.

TREATMENT

Multiple myeloma is usually treated by chemotherapy because there are drugs available which are sufficiently specific to damage malignant plasma cells before harming normal tissues. Where bone has been invaded by plasma cells, local radiotherapy is very beneficial in that it removes the malignant plasma cells and allows the bone to harden again. This prevents fracture and promotes healing where the bone has already cracked.

Cures are rare, but a temporary recovery can often be obtained by chemotherapy. Periodic examinations of the blood, the bone marrow and urine are essential to confirm the continued absence of diseased cells and abnormal proteins. Sometimes the recovery is only partial and one or more symptoms of myeloma persist throughout the prolonged treatment.

CANCER OF THE OESOPHAGUS

SYMPTOMS

The oesophagus is a muscular tube which connects the throat to the stomach. The first symptom of oesophageal cancer is difficulty in swallowing and usually the patient experiences food sticking somewhere behind the breast bone. It is solid food, particularly meat, which mostly causes this sticking sensation. If pain occurs it is generally felt as a burning sensation when food is swallowed and it also comes from behind the breast bone.

DIAGNOSIS

The diagnosis is established reasonably simply with the help of X-rays and a barium swallow, which outlines the abnormality in the oesophagus. It can be confirmed by *oesophagoscopy*, during which a slim instrument is passed through the mouth and throat into the oesophagus and through which the tumour can be directly viewed and a sample of tissue taken for examination under a microscope. It is sometimes helpful to wash the suspected area with a solution which is removed through the oesophagoscope. This solution is again examined for the existence of malignant cells which would have been shed by a small and so far invisible tumour.

TREATMENT

The treatment of cancer of the oesophagus is either by surgery or radio-therapy. Surgery is usually preferred when the cancer is limited to the lower part of the oesophagus. Radiotherapy can be used in conjunction with surgery or on its own. Its purpose is to shrink the cancer thereby relieving the difficulty in swallowing and easing the pain. After surgical removal of part of the oesophagus the remaining oesophageal stump is rejoined to the stomach. This usually means pulling up the stomach which in consequence reduces its capacity and may lead to bouts of indigestion after large meals. Total removal of the oesophagus which is a major surgical procedure is now only rarely performed.

OVARIAN CANCER

Ovarian cancer usually occurs after the change of life (menopause). If the growth metastasises, it usually travels through the lymphatic system rather than taking the bloodstream as its route.

SYMPTOMS

Lumps in the ovaries may cause no symptoms whatever and are usually first discovered on pelvic examination.

The only common sign, but rather a late one, associated with ovarian cancer, is enlargement of the abdomen. This is rarely due to the tumour itself but more often to accumulation of fluid in the abdomen produced by the presence of cancer. More rarely, abnormal vaginal bleeding occurs with ovarian cancer. Even less frequent symptoms are abdominal pain or a feeling of indigestion.

DIAGNOSIS

To confirm the diagnosis of ovarian cancer, an ultrasound examination may be performed which helps to locate any abnormal growth. It is carried out by an instrument which picks up the echoes of sound waves beamed into the body.

Outlining neighbouring organs, such as the intestine or kidneys, by the injection of a special dye or barium, will sometimes show compression of these structures by the ovarian tumour and so reveal its presence. It is useful at the same time to carry out a chest X-ray to exclude the possibility of ovarian metastases.

Further methods of establishing the diagnosis include insertion of a lighted instrument through a small peep-hole cut in the skin of the abdomen (*laparoscopy*), or opening the abdomen and having a look (*laparotomy*). This is carried out under a general anaesthetic and frequently a piece of the tumour is removed for biopsy.

TREATMENT

Treatment can consist of the removal of the tumour together with the ovary from which it arise, but such limited surgery is rare. More often both ovaries and the uterus are removed as a precautionary measure or because the tumour has already spread. After surgery either radio-therapy or chemotherapy, or both, may be given to treat any remaining cancer. After the completion of treatment periodic check-ups are essential to determine the progress and in particular to guard against a recurrence of the disease.

SUMMARY

While cancer of the ovary is less common, it is more dangerous by far than cancer of the uterus or cervix, because the ovaries lie deeper in the abdomen and are therefore not easy to reach for early diagnosis. It usually causes symptoms very late and as a result, is less curable than other tumours. Prior to treatment, a chest X-ray and an intravenous pyelogram (an X-ray of the kidney after intravenous injection of a dye which is excreted by the kidney) is routinely carried out to find out how far the disease has spread. When cancer cells fall off the surface of the ovary, which they often do, they spread throughout the abdominal cavity and may irritate its lining and cause fluid to be formed. This condition is called *ascites*; it is a common problem to which, so far, there is no answer.

CANCER OF THE PANCREAS

The pancreas lies behind the stomach. It is a lengthy organ with a head nestling in the loop of the small intestine on the right side, a body in its mid-section and a tail that is situated on the left side, just in front of the spine.

The pancreas has two functions; one is to release insulin and the other is to produce the pancreatic juice which contains enzymes that aid the digestion of food. This pancreatic juice is passed along the main pancreatic duct to enter the small intestine at the head of the pancreas. Most pancreatic tumours start in the cells of the pancreatic duct system and are more frequently situated in the head of the pancreas than in the body or tail.

SYMPTOMS
The most common sign of pancreatic cancer is vague pain in the upper abdomen which spreads to the back. This pain may be worse after eating or when lying down and sometimes can be relieved by sitting up or leaning forward. If the growth arises in the head of the pancreas it may block the bile duct as it enters the intestine and cause jaundice, because bile is being retained in the liver instead of passing into the intestine.

DIAGNOSIS
The diagnosis of a pancreatic tumour while the growth is still reasonably small causes great difficulty, because this cannot be seen on ordinary X-ray pictures of the upper abdomen. It can only sometimes be outlined on a barium swallow, which may demonstrate a narrowing in the stomach or duodenum, caused by pressure from a pancreatic tumour. More recently, radioactive, CAT and ultrasound scanning have all been used to try to look at the interior of the body, by creating an image of the organ and examining its outline. These methods may eventually lead to an earlier diagnosis of pancreatic cancer, which like other cancers can only be firmly established by a positive biopsy.

TREATMENT
The only recognised treatment for pancreatic cancer is surgery but because of the depth of the pancreas in the upper abdomen and the difficulty in diagnosing it at an early stage, surgical results are very disappointing, as the tumour is usually inoperable by the time the diagnosis is made.

Palliative surgery has, however, an important place in the relief of symptoms due, for instance, to the blockage of the common bile duct as it enters the duodenum. This can be achieved with the help of a by-pass operation, thereby relieving the jaundice.

Neither radiotherapy nor chemotherapy have so far proved useful in the treatment of pancreatic cancer on account of their limited effectiveness.

CANCER OF THE PROSTATE

The prostate gland is located at the base of the penis, just below the bladder and in front of the rectum.

SYMPTOMS

Prostatic symptoms are usually caused by enlargement of the prostate and are very common in men over 40. Such enlargement can either be benign or malignant and the symptoms they cause vary from difficulty in urinating, to dribbling, or difficulty in holding back urine. Enlargement which blocks the free-flow of urine is usually benign (noncancerous) and the condition is relieved by surgical removal of part or of all the prostate.

Prostatic cancer, which can be treated either by surgery, radiotherapy or hormonal therapy, spreads readily outside the prostatic gland to the skeleton, in particular the pelvis and lower spine. It is only very rarely that cancer of the prostate develops without giving urinary difficulties, in which case the first sign of trouble may be low backache due to metastatic spread to the bone.

DIAGNOSIS

Cancer of the prostate is revealed on internal examination as a rather irregular and unusually firm area in the otherwise smooth, soft prostatic gland. Only a biopsy will clinch the diagnosis and establish whether or not the growth is malignant.

TREATMENT

It is not unusual for elderly patients to have cancerous cells present in the prostate. In most of these patients the disease is harmless and therefore no aggressive treatment may be necessary because the cancer is growing so slowly that it is unlikely to cause any complications or spread outside the gland.

In cases where the tumour has not spread but is actively growing, removal of the prostate is necessary. An alternative treatment is radiotherapy which attempts to destroy the growth by means of radiation.

The prognosis, as well as the patient's comfort and general condition, is determined by the eventual spread of cancer outside the prostatic gland. Very rarely this spread may occur at a time when rectal examination does not reveal any abnormality in the prostate.

Since the prostate is under hormonal control of *testosterone* produced in the testes, removal of the testes (*castration* or *orchidectomy*) sometimes influences the spread of the disease and may temporarily relieve the discomfort due to bone pain.

Cancer affecting other genital organs of the male, mainly the scrotum and penis is fortunately uncommon and usually treated by surgery or radiotherapy. More frequent is cancer of the testis, which will be described elsewhere.

CANCER OF THE SKIN

Most skin cancers begin in the epithelial cells of the skin. Skin has two layers: the top layer or *epidermis* and the underlying *dermis*. Cell division takes place in the deepest (basal) layer next to the dermis, and as cells die they are replaced by new ones.

The epidermis also contains pigment cells, called *melanocytes*, which produce the brown pigment *melanin* which is incorporated in the multiplying cells and which protects them from the damage caused by ultraviolet light. The rate of pigment production is accelerated when exposure to sunlight is increased; this is the process that produces a suntan and, when out of control, can cause a melanoma (skin cancer).

SYMPTOMS

Skin cancer has many different appearances. It may start as a small, pale, waxy lump that eventually bleeds and crusts. It occurs mainly on sun-exposed areas, such as face, scalp, neck, hands and arms.

Then there is the melanoma which usually, but not invariably, arises in a pre-existing mole or coloured skin-patch, present since birth. The surface is uneven, it is blackish or brown, or may be mottled with shades of red and blue. Sometimes the surrounding skin may become inflamed, red and tender. It can turn into an open sore that bleeds.

Skin cancer is sometimes preceded by rough red areas of skin, usually on the face, neck, hands or legs. They are called *actinic-keratoses* and do not always turn into cancer. The anti-cancer ointment 5 *fluorouracil* is very effective in dealing with this problem.

There are two common cancers of the skin and one less common and all three are usually induced by sunlight. The first is the *rodent ulcer* or *basal cell carcinoma* which arises in the basal cell layer, does not metastasise and is, therefore, readily curable. The second, *squamous carcinoma* is made up of squamous epithelium and can spread to regional lymph nodes. It is also readily curable.

Finally there is the melanoma, which arises in the skin's melanocytes and which has a tendency to spread and form distant matastases. Although still relatively rare, its incidence is steadily increasing all over the world, a high price to pay for vanity and the commands of fashion, in the form of a sun-tanned, bronzed body.

Melanoma can appear anywhere on the skin. On men it is most common on the head and neck, on women, the legs and feet. It can also begin in the eye, mouth, nose, vagina and anus.

Scandinavia now has 11 new cases of melanoma per 100,000 people each year and this figure is doubling every 10 years. Queensland, Arizona and New Mexico have 32 new cases per 100,000 and in Queensland this figure doubles every 15 years. In Arizona and New Mexico the incidence has quadrupled in the past 10 years and is entirely confined to the 'Anglo' population of North-European descent, sporting a fair complexion. Epidemiological evidence is building up to suggest that the rapidly increasing incidence of *cutaneous malignant melanoma* is related to greater exposure of white skin to strong, natural sunlight. The patient with a melanoma is, however, not the man or woman who has spent a lifetime in an outdoor occupation and who has a high total lifetime dose of natural sunlight. He or she is more at risk of developing one of the other two types of skin cancer. By contrast, the patient with melanoma is two to three decades younger and is most often an indoor office worker of high socio-economic state. There is a relationship between severe sunburn and development of melanoma in the following five years, suggesting that short periods of intense burning sunlight are a risk factor, as is exposure of areas other than face and hands, particularly in people who cannot tolerate ultraviolet light and freckle easily.

The sun emits an ultraviolet light B and, as is known, these rays produce a tan readily, but they burn first. Long-term exposure can cause premature skin ageing and tumours. The rays emitted by sunbeds are usually ultraviolet light A and these rays cause tanning without burning. So far no serious long-term effects have been reported and at this stage ultraviolet light A can be considered to be non-carcinogenic on its own. However, when used in conjunction with the sun's ultraviolet light B, it seems that ultraviolet light A, in regular use of sunbeds, may be able to increase ultraviolet light B's ability to promote development of non-melanoma skin-cancer, as well as of malignant melanoma.

The only advantage of sunbeds is the production of vitamin D in the skin, which of course is also available in the normal diet; otherwise lying on a sunbed, either in the short or long term is not a pastime to be encouraged.

When sun-bathing, a barrier sun-lotion or sun-cream should be used, so that one can sit safely in the direct sunlight, the harmful rays having been filtered out. The cream should be re-applied at frequent intervals, particularly after swimming or when sweating hard. It is well to remember that no barrier cream is completely effective in the southern hemisphere when the sun is strongest and you should be very careful in tropical countries. This also applies to high altitudes: the higher up the more forceful the sun. As snow reflects the sun, particular care of the skin is necessary when skiing. In any case, people who are prone to sunburn should always wear a hat and a long-sleeved shirt, especially on the beach.

TREATMENT
Surgical removal of a malignant skin lesion is a very effective method of treatment in all three types of skin cancer. In the case of a melanoma the surgeon, however, takes an even wider margin around and under-neath the tumour and sometimes even removes underlying muscle. A skin graft may have to be applied to cover the skin defect caused by the wide cut.

Where surgery is difficult or would leave an unsightly scar, radio-therapy can be used but only for a rodent ulcer or a squamous cell carcinoma. In these types of skin cancer, results of treatment are usually good. They are less so for melanoma, which frequently meta-stasise and thus become incurable.

SUMMARY AND SYMPTOMS
In summary, here is a list of risk-factors contributing to the develop-ment of a melanoma, which increase with age:

1. A family history of melanoma.
2. Having previously had a melanoma.
3. Sudden appearance of a mole in fair-skinned, fair-haired people with light-coloured eyes and a tendency to sunburn easily and tan with difficulty.
4. Brown birthmarks which deepen in colour, increase in size and thickness, become irregular in shape or start to bleed.
5. A previous blistering sunburn.
6. Outdoor recreational habits in sunny regions with lengthy exposure to the sun, particularly in people with indoor occupations.

CANCER OF THE SPINAL CORD

Being made up of similar tissue as the brain, spinal cord tumours are similar to brain tumours but are less frequent. Most of the tumours found there have spread from other parts of the body. Spinal cord tumours may stop messages passing along the nerves between brain and body in much the same way as injury to the spinal cord does.

SYMPTOMS

The most common symptoms are pain, loss of feeling and ability to move arms or legs, and sometimes paralysis on one side with loss of sensation on the other.

DIAGNOSIS

Spinal tumours are diagnosed by careful physical and X-ray examination of the affected segment. Sometimes the spinal fluid is taken for analysis.

TREATMENT

Surgery is the usual treatment method and prompt action may lessen or even prevent permanent effects from these tumours. Radiotherapy is sometimes used along with surgery.

CANCER OF THE STOMACH

The stomach is a sac-like organ between the end of the oesophagus and the small intestine.

SYMPTOMS

One of the first symptoms of stomach cancer is indigestion and for this reason it usually remains unnoticed. In some cases of cancer of the stomach, indigestion may be associated with the feeling of heartburn and slight nausea. Loss of appetite and mild stomach pains are also warning signs to be noted. Vomiting, weight loss and pain are late signs, as is blood in the stools which can be either red or black in colour.

DIAGNOSIS

Since pernicious anaemia often leads to stomach cancer, a blood test is urgently required when indigestion persists. So is a test for the amount of acid in the stomach, because lack of acid is frequently associated with stomach cancer. As already stated the stools must be examined for the presence of blood.

Since the stomach outline shows up clearly on X-ray examination of a contrast-filled stomach (barium meal), cancer of the stomach is usually diagnosed by this procedure. Further examinations include gastroscopy, when an instrument using a flexible tube with a light and a series of mirrors, is passed through the mouth and oesophagus into the stomach, and a biopsy.

TREATMENT

The standard treatment for cancer of the stomach is surgery which may mean removing part or all of the stomach. Following this, if indigestion and other difficulties are to be avoided, it will be advisable to eat several small meals every day, instead of having two large ones.

Both chemotherapy and radiotherapy have so far not made any worthwhile contribution to the treatment of stomach cancer and are therefore not used.

CANCER OF THE TESTIS

The testes or testicles are egg-shaped organs suspended below the penis in a pouch of skin called the scrotum.

SYMPTOMS

Cancer of the testes mainly affects young men and is easily detectable as a small hard lump about the size of a pea. In the early stages it is usually painless and gives no warning of the danger it represents. Being so easy to reach, the testicles should be subjected to regular examination by hand similar to the regular examination for breast cancer in women. Husbands and wives should be taught what it is they are looking for and should be encouraged to carry out such examinations on their partners at least once a month. Other later symptoms of testicular cancer include enlargement of the organ, a heavy feeling in a testicle, a sudden build up of fluid or even blood in the scrotum.

DIAGNOSIS

The diagnosis is confirmed by a biopsy and further help is the detection in the bloodstream of two substances, one called *alphafetoprotein* and the other *human chorionic gonadotropin*. The measurement of these proteins can be helpful not only in the diagnosis and the detection of spread of the disease but also in assessing the effectiveness of treatment and the discovery of a recurrence.

Once the diagnosis has been made an X-ray of the chest is taken to ensure there is no secondary growth in the lungs. An intravenous pyelogram is carried out and a *lymphangiography* is ordered to show up involvement of lymph nodes. This involves injection of a dye between the toes which will travel up the legs and outline lymphatics and enlarged lymph nodes on the X-ray. Finally, a CAT scan is used to confirm or exclude the presence of enlarged lymph nodes.

TREATMENT

The treatment for testicular tumour is a combined one and can involve surgery, radiotherapy and chemotherapy. The first step always includes surgical removal of the affected testicle. If all the additional investigations have proved to be negative this may be the only treatment required. Usually it is thought safer to follow orchidectomy (removal of the testis) with a full course of post-operative radiotherapy aimed at all lymphatic channels.

There are two main groups of tumours affecting the testes: the *seminoma* and the *teratoma*. Of these, the seminoma has a much more favourable prognosis owing to its being so very radio-sensitive and therefore readily responsive to radiotherapy alone. In the case of teratoma extra chemotherapy is recommended.

Having a testis removed does not involve any 'loss of manhood' and a patient is rendered neither sterile nor impotent. One healthy testis is enough for full sexual function. Following treatment it is imperative to have regular check-ups and to test for the presence of either of the two proteins in the bloodstream.

CANCER OF THE UTERUS

The womb, also called the uterus, is pear-shaped. The upper, broader part is called the body and the lower end, which opens in the vagina, is the cervix. Both parts can be affected by cancer and in each case the symptoms, the treatment and the prognosis are similar.

The body of the uterus is frequently the site of benign tumours, often called fibroids. They do not invade surrounding tissues or spread to other organs, but when they press against normal tissues they can cause pain or bleeding and for this reason may require surgical removal. After the normal menopause, uterine fibroids sometimes become smaller and may even disappear. This is not so with cancer arising either in the body of the uterus or in the cervix.

SYMPTOMS OF CERVICAL CANCER
The most common symptom of cervical cancer is bleeding between periods or bleeding on intercourse. Sometimes there is only an increased vaginal discharge.

DIAGNOSIS
All these symptoms are warning signals which require vaginal examination by a doctor. Such examination involves examination by hand and the insertion of a small duck-bill instrument called a *speculum*, which allows inspection of the cervix and of the upper vagina. This enables the doctor to take a cervical smear with a wooden spatula, a test that is painless and very quick. The sample of cells collected from the cervix can then be checked. If there are any abnormalities, bigger samples of tissue are removed from suspect areas of the cervix at another examination.

The presence of atypical cells (also called *dysplasia*) is a pre-cancerous condition. When left untreated it may advance to *carcinoma in situ*, a cancer inside the layer of cells where it began. This is the earliest stage of malignancy that can be detected.

TREATMENT
There are two main forms of treatment for cervical cancer depending in particular on the stage of advancement of the disease but also on the patient's age and general condition. Surgery is recommended only for the early stages and involves the partial removal of the cervix for carcinoma in situ and hysterectomy (womb removal) for the more advanced yet still localised growth.

Radiotherapy is the alternative. It usually consists of insertion of caesium into the vaginal vault and inside the uterine canal. This is given in three treatments, each lasting for 24 hours and given at weekly intervals. The treatment is combined with external ray treatment to the pelvic side-walls, in order to treat the regional lymph nodes, to which the disease frequently spreads at an early date. Such treatment is usually given on an outpatient basis over several weeks.

Neither treatment causes any actual pain but unpleasant side-effects such as diarrhoea, frequent urination and discomfort, though temporary, are common. They usually disappear within a few weeks after completion of treatment. Chemotherapy so far has little to offer in the treatment of cervical cancer.

SYMPTOMS OF CANCER OF THE BODY OF THE UTERUS

The first symptom of cancer of the body of the uterus is abnormal bleeding from the uterus. It usually occurs after the menopause and is the most common symptom of *endometrial* cancer (the lining of the uterine body is called *endometrium* and this is where the cancer arises).

DIAGNOSIS

Menstrual bleeding after regular menstruation has stopped should not be considered to be part of the change of life. It should always be reported to a doctor and investigated, often by *dilatation and curettage* (commonly called a D and C). This is usually carried out under anaesthesia and involves expanding the cervix enough (dilatation) to permit insertion of a small instrument which removes material from the uterine lining (curettage). The procedure does not take more than ten minutes and examination of the removed specimen will establish the presence or absence of malignancy beyond doubt.

TREATMENT

The standard treatment for endometrial cancer consists of a preliminary insertion of a radiation source (radium or caesium) into the cavity of the uterine body for 24–48 hours and surgical removal of the entire womb, called total hysterectomy. Post-operative radiation is usually not given but may become necessary in the case of extensive spread of the disease.

Uterine cancer has been found to be sensitive to the female hormone progesterone and hormone treatment is employed in cases where the disease has recurred after surgery or radiation therapy.

4·CANCER IN CHILDREN

Only accidents claim more lives among children than cancer. These cancers are very malignant and, unless treated early, preferably by a team of consultants in a large centre specialising in childhood cancer, are rapidly fatal.

The more frequent childhood cancers include Wilms' tumour, neuroblastoma, Ewing's sarcoma, rhabdomyosarcoma, osteogenic sarcoma and, of course, acute lymphoblastic leukaemia.

All three forms of treatment, surgery, radiotherapy and chemotherapy, are employed, singly or in combination, and great advances have been made in the management of the disease.

One of the reasons why such treatment is best carried out in large centres is the availability of adequate equipment and the presence of medical staff specially trained to select the most effective combination of treatments currently used. Another reason is the expertise of the nursing staff in providing sympathetic psychological support for grieving parents and relatives faced with the possibility of their children actually dying.

There are two fundamental differences between cancers in adults and those occurring in children. First, only a few organs in the body are affected by childhood cancer and these are not usually the ones involving cancer in adults. Second, more than 90 per cent of childhood cancers are sarcomas, whereas in adults carcinomas are much more common.

The sarcomas usually grow with great speed and metastasise widely to other parts of the body quite early. Without prompt treatment survival tends to be short; over half these children die of the disease.

However, the reason why many forms of childhood cancer can be cured, springs from the fact that they consist of rapidly growing tumour cells which respond to anti-cancer drugs as well as being sensitive to damage by radiation.

Adjuvant chemotherapy, that is drug treatment for assumed but unproven micro-metastases after surgery or radiotherapy, has greatly increased the cure rate in Wilms' tumour, osteogenic sarcoma, Ewing's sarcoma and rhabdomyosarcoma, something so far not achieved in cancers occurring in adults.

COPING WITH CHILDHOOD CANCER

There probably is no situation more agonising for parents to face than the prospect of a child dying of cancer. Other children in the family may also find it difficult to handle the child's illness emotionally, sometimes more so than the sick child.

As a direct result, divorces are common among parents of these children, and brothers and sisters frequently resent the attention the parents give to the sick child at their expense. In addition, the family may also have to face economic hardship as a result of the child's illness, if one parent has had to give up a job to nurse him. No family can cope with a financial crisis and such psychological difficulties at the same time without support from outside.

Medical centres routinely treating children offer many services to help the family to cope with this stressful situation. In particular they set up discussion groups between parents so that an exchange of views of common problems can take place and fears about the death of their child can be shared. The mere fact that other parents have to face similar problems is very consoling. Similarly children in hospital can discuss their illness with other children. It helps them face their disease and encourages them to talk about it with their parents without having to be afraid of upsetting them. It is so much easier when neither parents nor the child need to hide their fear of death from each other. Above all, what is most important is for parents to ensure that the child continues to feel part of the family.

ACUTE LYMPHOBLASTIC LEUKAEMIA

Acute lymphoblastic leukaemia or ALL, as it is usually called, affects children between the ages of two and seven and rarely after fifteen. Leukaemia is a generalised disorder of the bone marrow, which is where white blood cells come from. It is in this spongy network of tissue which fills up the cavities of the bones that the uncontrolled reproduction of white cells takes place in leukaemia. What it is that produces the leukaemia remains unknown; it does not seem to be related to a child's health or diet.

SYMPTOMS

One of the key points of leukaemia is the increased reproduction of the white cells which replicate in such numbers as to swamp the bone marrow, and so interfere with the development of normal cells in the bone marrow. The resulting decrease, particularly in the normal red cells, is responsible for many of the symptoms of leukaemia. Therefore, one of the first signs will be anaemia, which shows that the number of red blood cells has decreased. As a result, the child will be very pale and have much less energy than usual. The other bone marrow cells whose numbers are usually decreased are the platelets. When these cells are severely reduced in numbers, they may make the patient prone to spontaneous bleeding and excessive bruising. Another symptom is that the child is more open to infection, because of the poor quality of the rapidly dividing white cells, which are unable to defend the body against disease-producing organisms.

DIAGNOSIS

An early diagnosis of childhood leukaemia is very difficult because the signs are the same as those of many other minor illnesses through which children always seem to be passing and which are generally treated at home without medical help. No blame can possibly be attached to parents for any delay in taking their child to the doctor for diagnosis. The suggestion that had the child received treatment sooner, the severity of the disease might have been lessened or the child might even have been cured, is incorrect because the long-term response to therapy in childhood leukaemia is not clearly affected by how early the disease is diagnosed. Eventually the diagnosis is made by a simple blood test, which will reveal the true nature of the disease. It is confirmed by removing some tissue from the bone marrow and examining it under a microscope.

TREATMENT

Acute lymphoblastic leukaemia in children is no longer an incurable disease as a result of the vast progress made in chemotherapy in the past 20 years. Multiple drugs are used simultaneously, the main idea being that, whereas the cancer-destroying effect of the various drugs will be cumulative, each of these drugs will have different but mild side-effects, which will make them much more tolerable. An important feature of this drug treatment is the reduction of the dose of each of these drugs, which will prevent permanent damage to normal tissues.

The price of a cure for a child receiving chemotherapy is a very high one in terms of side-effects. Loss of hair, though temporary, can be very traumatic to a child attending school, because he may become the target of cruel comments from other children. The feeling of tiredness, nausea and vomiting, with total lack of appetite, is also very hard for a child to bear.

The parents' burden is a heavy one, because of the agony associated with seeing one's child suffer as a result of the treatment, and with regard to the uncertainty of the prognosis. They will also have to make a very difficult decision if the disease affects a boy. It has been found that the leukaemic cells use the boy's testes as a sanctuary from where, after months or years, a re-infection may occur. This discovery was made as a result of the vastly superior cure rates in girls than in boys.

To eradicate the disease from the testes, X-ray therapy is used which, of course, will sterilise the irradiated boy for life, meaning that although he will not be impotent and should be able to develop most of the male secondary characteristics and can lead a normal sexual life, he will be infertile and not able to have children of his own. This is a hard decision which parents have to make on behalf of a boy usually only 7–12 years old.

Twenty years ago most children died within a month of the diagnosis. Nowadays 70 per cent of children will live five years and 50 per cent of these are eventually cured, but the combined course of treatment lasts about four years.

Treatment is given in three stages. During the first stage the blood returns to normal. However, the disease may still be present in the brain, spinal cord and testes. Treatment to the brain and testes is usually given by means of radiotherapy, whereas the spinal cord is treated by chemotherapy when the drug is directly injected into the spinal canal during the second stage of treatment. This protective phase is directed at the central nervous system because, as mentioned before, it so frequently offers sanctuary to leukaemic cells. Finally, in the third stage, *maintenance* drug therapy is carried out for two to four years.

The two drugs usually used in the first stage of treatment are *vincristine* and *predinsone*. Vincristine is given once a week by injection, whereas predinsone is taken orally in pill-form, several times a day. Vincristine can cause nerve damage resulting in a feeling of tingling mainly in hands and feet. Predinsone increases the appetite and leads to puffiness of face, which is sometimes described as 'moonface', but these changes are only temporary.

By the end of one month's treatment of ALL, the blood test results usually return to normal and the bone marrow appears free of leukaemic cells.

In the second stage, methotrexate is injected directly into the spinal canal. This spinal puncture, carried out under local anaesthetic, is not actually painful, but it can be somewhat unpleasant. Radiation to the head is quite free of bothersome side-effects except, of course, for the temporary loss of hair.

The maintenance therapy can last up to four years. The drugs, usually given by mouth during this period, are in such moderate doses that they rarely cause any noticeable side-effects. The only upsetting aspect of treatment during this final, though long phase, is the bone-marrow examination needed every two months to check for signs of a relapse.

At the end of these three or four years of treatment, all chemotherapy is stopped, provided that the leukaemia has not recurred. After this the child will be monitored by means of blood tests and/or bone marrow punctures at three to six month intervals.

The chances of a permanent cure following this treatment are excellent. During treatment, the child is much more liable to contract a sore throat, a cold, flu, a cough or other infections, because the immune defence system is depleted, as a result of the effects of the drugs on the white cells. Early treatment of such infections is necessary, because the child becomes very sick with these everyday infections that would not really affect a healthy child at all. Chickenpox in a child with acute leukaemia is particularly hazardous, because it can cause fatal pneumonia.

Parents of children with acute leukaemia must always live in fear that their child will contract one of the childhood illnesses and die. The compromise between being over-protective and isolating the child from friends and school-mates and allowing him to lead a near normal life is a difficult one for the parents to get absolutely right.

The prognosis in children developing recurrent leukaemia is an unfavourable one. In these serious cases, a bone marrow transplant may have to be considered because it may save about 10 per cent of these children even after the disease has recurred.

It must, however, be remembered by all concerned that a bone marrow transplant is a hazardous procedure which involves whole body irradiation (or a large dose of drugs), which is used to destroy all bone marrow cells, a procedure which can be associated with particularly unpleasant nausea and vomiting. To be successful, normal marrow from a brother or sister has to be transplanted into the sick child's marrow, where it will grow and produce all the various types of normal blood cells. However, unless the donor is an identical twin, these cells will differ from those of the patient. As a result they will be recognised as foreign by the body's immune system and cause a mostly fatal graft-versus-host disease, which damages organs such as the skin, the gastro-intestinal tract and the lungs. The chances of a permanent recovery are only about 50 per cent and are best when the transplant occurs before the disease recurs.

Although the cure rate of ALL continues to improve, a number of children will inevitably die of the disease. When this happens, it is important for the parents to feel, looking back, that they have tried all known treatments and that they had made their sick child's last few years as comfortable and as enjoyable as was possible. They will always think of him, they will always miss him and they may often cry for him, but they will never have reason to reproach themselves for not having tried harder.

In a recent review of the psychological consequences of childhood leukaemia it was found that 20–30 per cent of parents required psychiatric treatment (mainly for anxiety and depression), that 25 per cent of mothers experienced chronic sexual difficulties and that 20 per cent of parents had serious matrimonial disharmony: such is the emotional burden borne by the anxious relatives of a child with cancer.

EWING'S SARCOMA

Ewing's sarcoma is extremely malignant. By the time it is discovered, metastasis has already occurred in 90 per cent of children. The favourite site is the thigh bone (femur), also the pelvic bones and shoulder. It occurs most frequently between the ages of five and sixteen. The first symptom is usually a painful swelling of the bone. The diagnosis is, as always, confirmed by a biopsy.

TREATMENT

The treatment consists of radiotherapy and chemotherapy. Radiation is used to remove the tumour locally at its original site and chemotherapy is employed to treat the metastases present in most children. Without it, up to 85 per cent of children have a recurrence at a distant site, mainly in the lungs, liver and other bones.

OSTEOGENIC SARCOMA
Osteogenic sarcoma commonly arises in boys between the ages of 10 and 25 years. The femur (thigh bone) and the tibia (shin bone) are the favourite sites; it also occurs in the humerous (bone of the upper arm).

SYMPTOMS
The first symptom again is a painful bone swelling and again it is stressed that any bone pain in a child lasting longer than one week should be investigated. Before chemotherapy was introduced, 85 per cent of children with an osteosarcoma died within two years of amputation of the limb affected by the cancer.

DIAGNOSIS
The diagnosis is usually made on X-raying the affected limb and then confirmed by biopsy. By the time the diagnosis is made the tumour has already metastasised, usually to the lungs and though they may be undetectable at the time, these microscopic deposits will continue to grow and eventually kill the child, even if the entire cancer is removed by amputation.

TREATMENT
With the addition of chemotherapy the cure rate, which used to be 15 per cent by amputation alone, has risen, as in the case of most child-hood cancers, to roughly 50 per cent.

A child that has lost a limb due to amputation will require intensive rehabilitation. This is usually available at all larger centres dealing with childhood cancer.

WILMS' TUMOUR
Wilms' tumour is a tumour of the kidney in a child. It accounts for about 7 per cent of all cancer in children. The tumour usually develops before the age of four and certainly before the age of eight. The tumour grows to a great size very rapidly and may weigh up to 10 lb (4.5 kg) at the time of discovery. Parents who think that their child's abdomen is swollen and note that the swelling persists for several days, should consult a doctor.

DIAGNOSIS

The diagnosis is made by means of an intravenous pyelogram. Chest X-rays and a bone and liver scan will reveal the extent of spread to other organs.

TREATMENT

The treatment of Wilms' tumour consists of a combination of surgery, radiotherapy and chemotherapy. In very young children surgery, followed by chemotherapy to kill cancer cells which have spread to other parts of the body, may be enough without using radiotherapy as well. Approximately 80 per cent of all children with Wilms' tumour are cured by this combined approach.

NEUROBLASTOMA

Neuroblastoma is another highly malignant tumour which mostly occurs in infants; about 80 per cent occur in children under five. It arises from remains of embryonic tissue mostly in the abdomen and invades surrounding tissues and distant organs. The first symptom is usually an abdominal swelling or excessive sweating due to the secretion of special hormones called *catecholamines*.

DIAGNOSIS

The diagnosis is usually made by an X-ray which reveals an abdominal mass with calcifications, possibly in conjunction with breakdown products of catecholamines in the child's urine.

Age is an important factor in prognosis. At birth an infant with neuroblastoma has almost a 100 per cent chance of being cured; over the age of one that chance drops to 50 per cent and a child older than two probably only has a 20 per cent chance of cure. The reason for this age dependence is the lower malignancy of the tumour in a small baby which usually is localised and can be removed.

TREATMENT

Neuroblastoma is much harder to cure than Wilms' tumour because it is usually very widespread on discovery and is not so responsive to chemotherapy. The over all cure rate is about 30 per cent, with young children doing best. One intriguing feature about neuroblastoma in the very young is its tendency to *spontaneous regression*, even when it is quite widespread.

RHABDOMYOSARCOMA

SYMPTOMS
This type of cancer can arise anywhere in the body and the symptoms will depend on the site where it develops; in a muscle it looks like a bruise or in the nose like a bloody polyp. However, if a lump persists, it always deserves attention.

TREATMENT
Rhabdomyosarcoma arises from immature muscle. It is a highly malignant tumour but quite remarkable progress in its treatment has resulted from adjuvant chemotherapy. New drugs are administered after the original mass has been removed by surgery and irradiation by radiotherapy. The number of children cured has risen from a mere 15 per cent to 50 per cent.

Treatment should of course be carried out at a major centre dealing with childhood cancer. The results of treatment are best in cases where a localised tumour could be completely removed; about 80 per cent of these children are cured, whereas only 10 per cent of children who have widespread disease live more than two years.

5·CANCER-CAUSING FACTORS

Most of the advances in our knowledge of cancer-causing factors come from recent epidemiological studies. Epidemiology (a term coined by Hippocrates in 40 BC) is the branch of medical science studying the causes and distribution of a disease in a people or community. In all, about 40 different factors have been found to be contributory causes of the more common forms of cancer in man. Some of these, such as pollution or industrial chemicals and their effluents, are man-made and their toxic effects can be controlled by strict regulations. Others such as diet, alcohol consumption, smoking or sexual habits, are more personal and cannot be controlled in this way. Because their nature and exact identity is not yet generally understood, they can cause a great deal of unnecessary anxiety among the less well-informed.

People are not only over-anxious about cancer, they are also extremely gullible. Some start suspecting the presence of cancer-causing compounds even in their surroundings: in the air, water or their food. Many people are influenced by newspaper and television reports and fear a number of unfounded trivial risks, while ignoring less sensational but nevertheless real, scientifically established causes. The identification of such high-risk causes is the end result of careful observation which has pinpointed, for instance, an unusually high death rate from either a specific cause or among a particular group of individuals. These carcinogenic factors can be divided into two groups: the *external* or environmental oncs and the *intrinsic* or genetic ones.

ENVIRONMENTAL FACTORS

What recent epidemiological findings have clearly shown is that when we look at the distribution of cancer mortality world-wide, we can arrive at a number of very useful practical conclusions and some of them are quite surprising. There are, for instance, high and low-cancer

69

risk populations in the world and having insufficient food actually *reduces* the incidence of certain forms of cancer. Of even more practical interest, and very reassuring in view of the misleading, almost hysterical publicity on the subject, is the realisation that at present, food additives, insecticides, herbicides and pesticides cannot play anything but a very minor role in the development of cancer. Similarly, chemicals and other contaminants seem of minor impact in comparison with the importance of what we actually eat. What can be concluded from all this is that since our environment is under human control we should be able to manipulate it in a way which will lead to a reduction of cancer.

Epidemiologists have been able to identify people in different parts of the world who are more likely to contract cancer. Stomach cancer was found to be highest in Japan, liver cancer in East Africa, cervical cancer in Colombia and Puerto Rico, and breast and bowel cancer in all affluent Western countries. Identification of these clues allows recommendations which, if followed, should lower these high rates of specific forms of cancer. These clues pointed to numerous factors, including the effects of hormones, of chronic irritation or inflammation, of ageing, and of the impact of stress or one's emotional and psychological state. However, over half of the more common forms of cancer are related to *diet*, which makes the combined effect of food and drink a more important determinant of the risk of contracting cancer than even smoking.

THE FOOD WE EAT

Each item of food we allow to pass our lips throughout the day should therefore have been chosen with serious deliberation. This means that we must try to be consistently firm about the food we accept and the food we feel obliged to refuse.

By being careful about what and how much we eat we can reduce the probability of contracting one or more of the five killer diseases (heart disease, high blood pressure, strokes, diabetes and cancer), resulting from our greed and affluence, and from which less privileged nations do not generally suffer. In this context it surely is ironic that many Third World communities, so far not affected by the degenerative illnesses of the sophisticated West, should strive so desperately for greater affluence, which will bring in its wake the same toll of Western ill health!

There is a strikingly direct relationship between fat consumption and both breast and bowel cancer, which is reflected in the wide variation of these cancers between affluent and under-privileged nations. This variation tells us that with a suitable change in life-style, these common cancers should be avoidable in 80 per cent of cases. It is our incredibly short-sighted reluctance to break the habits of a lifetime which make such a life-saving improvement unlikely for many years to come.

CHEMICALS

Among the external cancer-causing factors there are also many chemical agents responsible for certain forms of cancer in the industrialised West.

Tobacco, particularly cigarette smoking, provides a sadly topical example of the role of such external factors. Lung cancer was half as common 40 years ago, when we smoked less, so we do know what to do to reduce it. Yet in a vast controlled study into the cause of lung cancer, Western societies are using themselves as experimental animals and sacrificing several million people in the process, instead of simply giving up smoking and reducing the possibility of this disease.

Some of these chemical agents actually interact with others to produce much greater effects. For example, British lung cancer incidence in non-smoking town dwellers and non-smoking country dwellers was found to be similar. But among smokers, lung cancer mortality in large towns was twice that in rural areas, presumably as a result of interaction between smoking and air pollutants. Similarly, such raised lung cancer incidence also occurs in asbestos workers who smoke, while asbestos workers who do not smoke tend to get asbestosis, a chronic lung disease rather than lung cancer.

In smokers who drink alcohol, the interaction between smoking and alcohol leads to a higher incidence of cancer of upper digestive and respiratory passages, probably the result of damage to the cell-lining covering these passages.

In Egypt, the combination of schistosomiasis (a parasitic bladder infection) and smoking is likely to cause bladder cancer.

GENETIC FACTORS

Compared with the very important role of these external (environmental) agents, the influence of intrinsic (genetic) factors in carcinogenesis pales into insignificance. Heredity (familial predisposition) plays only a minor role in cancer of the stomach, intestine, lung and breast. This will be dealt with in the appropriate section later, but let us now make some general observations on heredity.

When we are dealing with family susceptibility the important question to ask is whether the disease is actually due to some altered genetic pattern, or whether it is not much more likely that it is caused by environmental factors such as life-style or eating habits which affect all members of the family. Equally important is the question: which factor is more significant, the environmental or the genetic one? The answer, from the point of view of prevention, is that the environmental factors must be more important, because they are under our control, whereas the genetic factors are not. To give a practical example: fair-skinned, blue-eyed people are genetically pre-disposed to skin cancer on excessive exposure to ultraviolet sunlight. Although we can't change our skin, we *can* control our amount of exposure to sunlight!

It stands to reason that each one of us should be on the look-out for factors within our own control, which might promote such risks and try to avoid them. For instance, even light smokers, whose parents have lung cancer, run a fifteen-fold increase in risk of developing a lung tumour.

OTHER CANCER-CAUSING FACTORS

Apart from this type of inherited proneness to cancer (which, as stated, plays only an insignificant role in the general incidence of cancer), there is another kind which is started by a pre-existing illness. Examples include ulcerative colitis, which may lead to bowel cancer, pernicious anaemia which may lead to stomach cancer, and a special type of anaemia (called the Plummer Vinson syndrome) which is caused in thin frail, elderly women by a diet poor in iron and which usually culminates in throat cancer.

It is worth noting that in these cases cancer can mostly be prevented by dealing with the original disease. This has been dramatically demonstrated quite recently in tropical liver cancer. A fungus called *Aspergillus flavus* produces, under humid tropical conditions, a cancer-causing mould called aflatoxin which can contaminate groundnuts and grain if stored in unsatisfactory conditions. When these contaminated peanuts are eaten by people who have been previously infected by the hepatitis B virus, they will develop liver cancer in large numbers. Such outbreaks occur mainly in the under-privileged nations of East Africa, where storage facilities still remain very primitive.

Infection with the hepatitis B virus is probably the commonest cause of liver disease worldwide. There are over 200 million people with this infection, of whom many will die from liver damage, including liver cancer.

Preventing the virus-induced hepatitis B by means of vaccination has only just become possible and it protects the liver against cancer. There is now real hope that this infection and the disease it causes will eventually be wiped out for good.

Most of the identified industrial cancer-causing substances have operated over at least ten years before being discovered. During this long period the interaction between two mutagens, like smoking and asbestos, occurs. Smoking is the initiator that induces the early stages while asbestos is the promoter which acts on the later steps.

Similarly, smoking will promote upper respiratory and digestive tract cancer in habitual alcohol consumers; or cervical cancer in women with previous herpes genitalis and/or human papilloma virus infections; or bladder cancer in Egyptians with a parasitic bladder infection.

This two-stage progression in the development of cancer offers a great opportunity for effective cancer prevention. By avoiding the known promoter, its triggering action on the actual malignant process can be blocked, thereby preventing the disease altogether.

6·NUTRITION-RELATED CANCER

World-wide epidemiological studies carried out in the past two decades suggest that up to 80 per cent of human cancers, in particular bowel cancer, stomach cancer, breast cancer and head and neck cancer, are induced by what we eat and drink. Cancer of the prostate and of the pancreas are also affected by dietary factors, but to a much lesser extent.

THE LARGE BOWEL

Cancer of the large bowel is found mostly in affluent, highly-developed countries and it is much more common in urban areas than in rural, sparsely populated districts in those countries. Furthermore, there seems to be a direct link between the consumption of meat and the frequency of bowel cancer. This disease is virtually unknown in Tibet and Thailand, where practically no meat is consumed. It occurs with moderate frequency in Japan and Chile, where modest amounts of meat are consumed, but the highest incidence of bowel cancer occurs in Scotland, Canada, New Zealand, Australia and the USA, which are countries with the largest meat consumption.

In 1985 130,000 cases of bowel and rectum cancer were diagnosed in the US, of which 65,000 died. A further piece of conclusive evidence about the link between diet and bowel cancer is provided by the US black population. American blacks have shown a dramatic increase in bowel cancer following the introduction of the Bill of Rights and their resulting affluence. This has raised their standard of living and has enabled them to copy the diet of whites, including daily consumption of large amounts of meat. The extremely high bowel cancer rate in American Negroes stands in marked contrast to negroes in Africa, among whom bowel cancer is virtually unknown.

Evidence to show lower incidence of bowel cancer because of a higher consumption of cereals, fruit and vegetables in their diet, is provided by

US Mormons and Seventh Day Adventists in California. Similar evidence also comes from other parts of the world. For instance, in India, the Parsees who eat a Western-style diet suffer from bowel cancer much more frequently than the general Hindu population.

Further very convincing evidence is provided by Japanese migrants who have settled in Hawaii or California and who, on adopting a Western-style diet, including large beef consumption, have shown a parallel rise in cancer of the large bowel after one generation.

What, therefore, has been shown by these studies is that it is not only high meat consumption but a diet low in vegetables, particularly cabbage, broccoli and Brussel sprouts, which appears to increase the likelihood of developing cancer of the colon.

Similarly, a high-fibre diet seems to have a protective effect as shown by the low incidence of bowel cancer in rural Africans, as well as in Israelis of Asian or African origin who eat fibre-rich food.

SUMMARY

World-wide studies have confirmed conclusively that a diet high in total fat and high in red meat, especially when it is also low in fibre, vegetables and the mineral selenium (p. 85), is associated with a significantly increased incidence of large-bowel cancer. The disease eventually develops in approximately 6 per cent of the American population, and six million Americans who are alive today will die of it.

THE STOMACH

Cancer of the stomach is known to occur more frequently in lower class Western males around the age of 55 years. The incidence of stomach cancer can be lowered by eating Western-type vegetables, such as lettuce, tomatoes, celery and corn, whereas eating Japanese-style salted, seasoned, spiced or cured food tends to raise the frequency of stomach cancer.

Nitrites and nitrates are chemical substances containing nitrogen which are present in human saliva. These substances have been shown to cause stomach cancer in experiments on animals. Their role in human cancer is a complex one, but they do not appear to increase the risk of stomach cancer in people, particularly when they are eaten together with fruit, vegetables and salads. It is thought that they are neutralised by the high Vitamin C content of these foods. This is one reason why fresh vegetables and fruit should be eaten throughout the year, rather than seasonally. It is worth repeating that a reduced salt-intake is beneficial as regards avoiding stomach cancer.

THE BREAST

Convincing epidemiological evidence is available to show that diet is one of the many contributory factors to breast cancer. In Western countries the incidence of breast cancer continues to rise after the menopause, whereas it remains the same in Japan. This difference is believed to be due to dietary practices in the high-risk countries of the West. This belief is reinforced by the increased incidence over the past 40 years of breast cancer in American blacks. This again is thought to be due to eating more of the rich food now available to them as the result of their improved earning capacity.

Similarly, the latter-day increase of breast cancer in Japanese women is thought to be related to the recent shift of the Japanese to a more Western-style diet with a particular increase in fat consumption. This is known to affect the hormones associated with breast tissue.

THE OESOPHAGUS

Alcohol and tobacco are known to interact and reinforce each other's detrimental effect in the production of cancer. Too much of both increases the risk proneness to oesophageal cancer. There are a number of oesophageal-cancer 'hot-spots' in Western Europe, North America and the wheat-eating (as opposed to the rice-eating) parts of China.

When alcohol intake is excessive it can destroy hunger, seriously depress appetite and interfere with absorption of nutrients, vitamins and minerals. This can lead to an unbalanced diet and nutritional deficiencies which give rise to cancer.

THE PANCREAS

High fat consumption and over-eating are associated with an increased incidence of cancer of the pancreas. It is this excessively rich type of diet which has been linked with the climbing rates of pancreatic cancer in the West, particularly among American Jews who eat food much richer in fat than Jews of Asian or African origin. Dietary fats are thought to create carcinogens in the bile and cause it to flow back into the pancreas.

THE PROSTATE

There is a marked difference, both geographic and racial, between Western countries (including the USA and Britain) where prostatic cancer is common, and Japan and Africa where it is rare, as well as between the US black and white population, where the incidence is greater among blacks. Yet African blacks have a much lower incidence than even American whites, which suggests that environment affects American blacks. An important factor appears to be population density, as there are fewer deaths from prostatic carcinoma in sparsely populated areas in the USA. When prostates in men who have died from other conditions are examined through a microscope, unsuspected cancer is found in about 45 per cent of all men over the age of 50, but it is only in affluent societies that they seem to develop into active malignant lesions. This is probably caused by increased hormone production, resulting from over eating.

There is an interesting scientific relationship parallel between the incidence of prostatic cancer and that of breast and colon cancer. When comparing the high- and low-risk areas in the world, the one striking difference was found to be the intake of fat. In the high-risk areas the intake is double (40 per cent of the total calorie intake) that of the low-risk regions (20 per cent of the total calorie intake). When comparing geographic areas in the United States in relation to their whole-milk and beef consumption (as a measure of the fat-intake of the respective populations) it is found that the north-central and mid-west areas, with the highest fat consumption also have the highest prostatic-cancer mortality rate.

Like breast cancer, prostatic cancer is hormone-dependent and any factor, such as diet, affecting hormonal secretion, also influences the frequency of prostatic cancer. It is interesting to note that, in fact, a vegetarian diet was found to lower the prostatic cancer rate, possibly because of a decreased overnight release of such hormones as testosterone.

OUR DAILY BREAD

Our life expectancy is longer now than it was 200 years ago. It is longer, not because we are healthier but because of our greatly improved public health measures, in particular:

1. vaccination against smallpox, tetanus, whooping cough, diphtheria and infantile paralysis
2. sterilisation of water supplies
3. compulsory pasteurisation of all milk.

In fact our health is worse and this is due, to a large extent, to our food which is richer, softer and sweeter than ever before. It is richer because we eat more fat; it is softer because it is processed and refined to a high degree and has lost its natural fibre content (together with other nutrients) and it is sweeter because our greatly increased consumption of sugar makes us prefer sweet foods, which manufacturers are very happy to supply.

We already know what eating habits cause cancer and so must realise that by changing these eating habits we could avoid cancer and that the choice is ours, even if we decide to do nothing about it. Just as we assume (wrongly) that it is normal for old people to lose their mobility and energy, to suffer from rheumatism, arthritis and chestiness, to become overweight and lose some of their mental alertness, so we accept (again wrongly) cancer and heart disease to be part of our normal lives today; they certainly are not normal and the evidence that they need not be is clear.

There are about 40 substances that we should eat for good health, but no longer do; instead we fill ourselves with refined, high-calorie food, rich in fat and sugar and, as a result of feeling full, leave out certain food items which the body cannot do without. Too few of us realise that eating what we like and eating healthily *are* compatible and that as food and health are so closely related, our choice of food also decides our state of health.

There are two main reasons for eating: firstly we provide the body with nutrients for tissue growth and repair; and secondly, we eat for fun, which is obviously the more pleasurable one of the two, although rarely healthy.

Since it is food we eat, not nutrients, we need to find out which of the three main types of food (proteins, fats and carbohydrates) are most required for good health.

PROTEINS

Proteins are the main body-building and repair foods. The most concentrated sources are found in meat, fish, cheese, milk, eggs, nuts and soya beans. Other, smaller sources of protein are wheat and pulses. The total daily protein requirement is only 45g (1½oz) and should represent no more than 10 per cent of our daily food intake.

FATS

Fats give long-term energy because they take longer to be digested and absorbed into the system. They are found in foods as visible fats like lard, suet, cooking fat, oil, butter, margarine, cream and fat on meat, and as invisible fats in milk, fatty meat, cheese and oily fish. Small quantities are even contained in cereals. Vegetables and fruit, apart from avocado pears and olives, contain a very small amount of fat. When chemically analysed, fats contain, as part of their make-up, substances known as fatty acids. These come in three types:

Saturated Fatty Acids
These are found mostly in foods of mainly animal origin. Over long periods, eating too much food containing saturated fatty acids tends to increase the blood cholesterol level. These fats are found in cream, cheese, milk fat, butter, meat fat, cooking fat, dripping, lard, suet, coconut and palm oils, cocoa and chocolate, and in hard and soft margarines which are not specifically polyunsaturated.

Mono-unsaturated Fatty Acids
These fats neither raise nor lower blood cholesterol levels. However, they do add to the total daily fat (and energy) intake, and foods containing them also have some saturated fatty acids as well. They are found in largest amounts in olive oil, peanut oil, olives, and avocado pears.

Polyunsaturated Fatty Acids
These tend to lower blood cholesterol levels. They are found in safflower, sunflower, corn and soya-bean oil. Polyunsaturated margarines are a convenient source of this type of fatty acid. However, even the highest polyunsaturated fats are only 72 per cent poly, the rest being mono and saturated fat.

Essential Fatty Acids
Three fats are referred to collectively as Vitamin F. Although required in only very small amounts, they are nevertheless essential to health (that is why they are called essential fatty acids or EFA). They must be supplied in such foods as milk, cheese, eggs, nuts, sunflower or corn oil, linseed or wheatgerm.

The total daily fat allowance should be below 20 per cent (not as at present, over 40 per cent) of the daily food intake, that is less than 50g (1½oz). For instance, butter is pure fat, as is margarine. Cheese is equally unhealthy, because it is concentrated fat. If women, in particular, continue eating it in anything but small amounts they might just as well spread it on their thighs, because sooner or later that is where it will surely end up! Low-fat cheese is better, but no cheese is best. Other whole-cream/milk products should also be struck off one's shopping list. In fact, anything with the word cream in it is better omitted: cream cheese, whipped cream, ice cream, cream soup, sour cream and so on. If we substitute the word fat for cream and call them fat cheese, whipped fat, ice fat, fat soup or sour fat, because that is what they all are, it may be easier to give them up. Mayonnaise is also bad; it is full of fat and salt; one tablespoon has the calories contained in two table-spoons of white sugar. On the other hand, low-fat yoghurt is a wonderful substitute for sour cream, for instance in a baked potato.

CHOLESTEROL

Cholesterol is a fat which is found in the blood. It is one of the main factors contributing to heart disease and as a fat also represents a cancer risk. It is manufactured in the body but it is also supplied in food; there are four food-groups:

1. Cholesterol-free: all plants, vegetables and their products.
2. Low cholesterol: skimmed milk and low-fat yoghurt.
3. Medium cholesterol: fish, lean meats, whole milk and cheese.
4. High cholesterol: all offal (such as heart, liver, brain, sweetbread), roes, shrimps, prawns, Stilton, Cheddar and egg yolk.

Red meat also contains a lot of hidden fat; veal is leaner; skinless chicken is better but fish is even healthier; like cheese, meat is best left out altogether. This also goes for fried food. Grill, steam, boil or bake instead.

CARBOHYDRATES

There are two groups of carbohydrates. Natural, also called complex, carbohydrates are known as the 'good guys'. The simple processed or refined carbohydrates like white sugar are the 'bad guys', and contain sugar in the form of sucrose.

The natural carbohydrates are fruit, vegetables and whole grain products such as bread, cereals, flour, potatoes, rice, maize and pasta. They convert slowly into blood sugar and supply us with vitamins, minerals and roughage; they are the desirable ones.

The 'bad guys', those in soft drinks, colas, white bread, and sugary cereals are empty calories with little nutritional value. They are rapidly converted into glucose in the blood; they cause sugar imbalances, they exhaust the pancreas and can eventually lead to diabetes. They include all forms of sugar, whether white, brown, raw, or Demerara, glucose, syrup, treacle, molasses, jam and marmalades and also honey (which contains fructose not sucrose). Fructose is also found naturally in all fruits and in this form is easier to digest without putting a strain on the pancreas.

OBESITY

Obesity is a pre-cancerous stage. Avoid obesity and you can avoid cancer. There is a direct link between opulence, overweight and the cancers of affluence.

Fats and sugar are the two 'high-calorie risk' food components in any diet; they are needed by the body solely as a source of energy for heavy physical work and for athletic pursuits. In the absence of such physical activities, too much fat and/or sugar taken regularly will inevitably lead to fat storage and weight gain. Fat has the highest calorie content per volume and eating butter and margarine, or constantly frying foods in cooking fats or oil, will greatly increase calorie consumption.

Each ¼lb (120g) packet of butter or margarine provides over 1,000 calories. Fat forms at least 40 per cent of the total calorie content of cakes, biscuits, pastries, puddings, potato crisps, peanuts, chocolate and chocolate-covered sweets, sauces, cream soups, salad cream, sausages, mayonnaise, beefburgers, most meats, all fried food, cream, eggs, whole milk and cheese.

Of the carbohydrates consumed, one-third is taken as sugar and half of this is used in tea or coffee and the rest in manufactured and cooked foods. Sugar should be reduced to the status of a condiment, not only on account of its calorie content but because together with fibre-deficiency, it alters the dominant type of colon bacteria, thus increasing the risk of cancer of colon and rectum.

Drinking a total of five cups of either tea or coffee a day, with two teaspoons of sugar in each cup, gives 225 empty calories; most people throw away 10 per cent of their daily calorie intake on non-food. Similarly, alcohol provides no nutrition – only calories. A percentage of these surplus calories, not needed to fuel the body with energy, is then stored as body fat and this is what makes people overweight.

To lose weight, the amount of dietary fat and sugar taken must be reduced. Reduction of the complex carbohydrates is not a good thing because fibre-rich starchy foods are an essential part of a complete, balanced, healthy diet. Most people are, or at least should be, aware that short-term rapid weight loss with rigorous diets depends on loss of body water (with glycogen and protein) not body fat. It takes months for many overweight people to lose the actual excess fat. A weight reduction of 2lb (1kg) per week is the maximum loss desirable for the majority of adults. After weight loss, the energy intake should be permanently adjusted in order to avoid regaining weight; this can be achieved by increasing consumption of wholemeal bread and whole-grain cereals (high-fibre content), vegetables and fruit. Food rich in fat (meat products and fried food) and those rich in sugar have to be restricted on a long-term basis.

BEHAVIOURAL SLIMMING
Behaviour slimming is based on the idea that overweight people wishing to slim need first to be told how to recognise what causes their current bad habits. Then they must be shown how to invent methods to overcome these problems and so establish new, better patterns of behaviour. Few obese people are aware, for example, that they eat a great part of their food while walking about the house doing other tasks. They need to become conscious of this so that they can regulate their eating pattern. Those who wish to slim should have meals in a setting where they can appreciate that they have had a meal, without other distractions. In this way snacks between meals can be avoided, because the routine for meals has to be followed at all times. Many people eat more when they are bored, tired or under stress, so slimmers should pay special attention to their eating habits at these times. A considerable effort is demanded of the slimmer and success depends on his or her dedication.

Adopting the 'restricted foods' type of diets is undesirable for healthy people though they may be necessary for patients with allergies or other abnormalities. The most effective and painless way to lose weight is first to choose an ideal weight for the rest of one's life, then to try and reduce one's diet by 200 calories a day, through a mixed diet of skimmed milk, whole-wheat grain, vegetables, poultry, fish, fruit and the *occasional* egg – a diet which ensures an adequate amount of all vitamins and minerals. If, additionally, another 300 calories a day can be lost in physical activity (an hour's brisk walking), this will lead to a total daily reduction of 500 calories and will result in a weekly loss of 500g (one pound) of fat.

Since it takes months to gain weight it cannot, despite claims to the contrary, be lost in a few days. The only solution is to learn new eating habits and to keep them for life. Perhaps the best rule of all to help achieve this is always: '*eat little of everything and not too much of anything*'. In health, as in all other worthwhile pursuits, quick short-cuts actually never stand a chance.

Yet, since hope springs eternal in the human breast and since people are even more gullible than usual when it comes to health or slimming, they will be only too willing to believe what they read about instant loss of weight and will try to buy hope, as if they were in a betting shop or on the stock exchange. Inevitably they will lose because, as with the other areas of our lives, most great achievements have to be earned the hard way.

MICRONUTRIENTS (Vitamins and Minerals)

VITAMINS

Most people have an adequate vitamin intake in their diet, sufficient to ensure good health, yet in the UK the annual over-the-counter-sales of packaged vitamins is estimated at over £45 million. Similar figures are found in other parts of the Western world too. Although vitamin supplements are rarely needed for normal adults, they should be considered for:

– people who rarely go into the sunlight
– people with a restrictive diet, such as vegetarians and other food faddists
– people with a poor intake, such as anorexics, depressives and alcoholics
– people of advanced years
– people, such as commercial travellers, who regularly eat in canteens and low-price cafes
– people who live on packaged and 'fast' junk food
– convalescents, expectant nursing mothers, infants, young children and adolescents.

Here are some concentrated sources of the five principal vitamins:
Vitamin A: liver, carrots, apricots, spinach and cheddar cheese
Vitamin B (complex): brewer's yeast, unpolished rice, wheatgerm, whole grains, liver, cheese, fish, yoghurt, nuts, pulses. The essential Vitamin B_{12} is required in tracer doses. Except for yeast and seaweed it exists almost exclusively in foods of animal origin such as liver, most meats, milk, eggs and cheese. For this reason vegetarians may experience deficiency.
Vitamin C: rose hip, fresh citrus fruits, cabbage, red and green peppers, fresh green leaf vegetables, strawberries and watercress. Nobel-prize Laureate Dr Linus Pauling recommends high doses to maintain the

immunological defence system.

Vitamin D: milk, cheese, cod liver oil, herrings.

Vitamin E: wheatgerm, whole wheat, almonds, peanuts.

MINERALS

All minerals essential for health are plentiful in a mixed diet and mineral deficiency, therefore, is rare. For example, in a well-balanced diet, calcium is found in milk and cheeses, phosphorus in all meat products and eggs, magnesium in bran and nuts, iron in red meat, liver, black treacle and baked beans and zinc in meat, offal and shellfish.

One of the main functions of minerals is to keep a perfect balance between many of the acid and alkaline elements in the body. Sodium, potassium, calcium, magnesium, manganese, iron and copper are alkaline and iodine, phosphorus, chloride and sulphur are of an acid producing nature, thus preventing an alkaline excess. Sodium probably plays the most important role in keeping a perfect balance between the acid and alkaline elements in the body. The desirable daily intake of sodium, usually in the form of ordinary salt (sodium chloride), should not exceed a quarter of a teaspoon (one teaspoon has more than 2 grams). There is nothing good about adding sodium to our foods, because it is already in almost everything we eat in larger quantities than we need; there is salt in mayonnaise, cottage cheese, soya sauce, tomato sauce and a long list of other foods.

FREE RADICALS

A free radical (sometimes also called an oxygen radical) is an atom or a group of atoms with an uneven electrical charge, meaning that these atoms have acquired one surplus electron as a result of oxidation and become extra-reactive and determined to combine with something else. Inside the body this something else is usually the DNA (the cell's genetic blueprint) from which, in order to complete themselves, the radicals steal an extra electron; this can set up a chain reaction during which more free radicals are produced. These are then available to damage more cells, thereby interfering with normal cell production and initiating a mutation – a change of chemistry and function – as a result of which the cells will start dividing abnormally, in an uncontrollable manner, which may ultimately culminate in a cancerous growth. If the oxidative process can be prevented there will be no atoms with surplus electrons and so no mutation.

Free radicals are formed by many normal reactions, such as the presence of oxygen peroxide, or the inhaling of oxygen. For example, unsaturated oils such as vegetable oils, which are particularly susceptible to free radical damage become rancid, especially when heated.

The body defends itself against free radicals by using the small molecules that protect cellular DNA from oxidative damage. The most important among these are the three vitamins: A, C and E. The reason, for example, that Vitamin A in carrots, and carotene-containing yellow, red and green vegetables, provides effective protection against lung cancer in smokers, may be related to the high level of oxidants in both cigarette-smoke and tar, and how these are attacked by the carotene.

SELENIUM

Alternatively, there are enzymes designed to disarm free radicals. One such anti-oxidant enzyme is called *glutathione peroxidase* (GP). Its effective action depends on the mineral *selenium*. When the dietary intake of selenium is increased by a factor of ten the activity of GP will be doubled. In a number of studies it was found that people with a very low selenium level had a greater chance of getting cancer than those with a very high level. Similarly, breast cancer rates in selenium-rich parts of the world are unusually low.

Too little dietary selenium is associated with an increased risk of fatal cancer. What is more, low Vitamin E intake may enhance this effect. Selenium is abundant in meats, seafood, yeast, eggs, liver, kidney, garlic, onions and mushrooms. It is absent from refined foods, but ample supplies always exist in a balanced mixed diet. An adequate daily dose is 300 micrograms.

URIC ACID

Another anti-oxidant is uric acid. Its high blood concentration can be further increased by consumption of dietary *purins*, but too much can cause gout. Foods high in purins are sweet-breads, anchovies, sardines, shrimps, mackerel, liver, kidney, meat extracts and dried legumes. (In smokers a low uric acid concentration may represent a contributory factor to lung cancer.)

SUMMARY

Vitamin A, Vitamin C, Vitamin E, selenium and uric acid have been shown to be the most important anti-carcinogenic protective factors in our diet. Of these only selenium and uric acid are toxic in too high concentrations.

OTHER MINERALS

NITRATES
A great deal has been written about the danger from nitrites and nitrates used against the deadly botulism in the preparation of bacon and the curing of various meats, because in the body they combine with amines to produce nitrosamines, which are known to be strong carcinogens in most animals. Of course, traces of nitrosamines are found in both bacon and some processed meats but traces are also found in most vegetables such as spinach, radishes, celery, lettuce and turnips. In any case, nitrites are also found in human saliva and it is therefore not surprising that there is no evidence that in humans nitrite-treated foods are carcinogenic.

CYCLAMATES
As regards cyclamates, even in animals, more recent repeat-tests have failed to confirm the development of bladder tumours, following the original scare in the USA in 1969, when eight out of 240 rats on very high doses of cyclamates developed what appeared to be bladder tumours, four of which were subsequently confirmed as carcinomas.

SACCHARIN
Similarly, saccharin appears to be quite safe. It has been in use for 81 years and although three out of 100 rats fed huge amounts of saccharin developed bladder tumours when the experiment was first carried out in Canada in 1977 (resulting in the banning of saccharin in Canada), the results of these experiments have not since been confirmed by other experiments.

In any case, most epidemiological studies in humans since 1977 have failed to show any relationship between taking saccharin and bladder cancer. Significantly, diabetics have a lower bladder cancer incidence than that found in the rest of the population, possibly also because diabetics smoke less heavily than average.

There is, therefore, no evidence that artificial sweeteners such as cyclamates and saccharin cause cancer in man, and they should both be considered safe.

COOKING

During cooking, the outside of food can be burnt, for instance on charcoal grilling of steaks at barbecues, or when carbohydrates are caramelised, as on the brown-crust of toasted bread. These burnt or caramelised surfaces contain a large variety of DNA-damaging agents, which are *presumptive carcinogens*, known to produce cancer in animals. Good cooks do not usually burn much of the food they are cooking, but they do caramelise it.

The total amount of such burnt material consumed may be as much as several grams, a menacingly large amount when compared with a mere half-gram of burnt material inhaled in a single day by a person smoking 20 cigarettes, and who as a direct result, can expect a shortening of his or her life expectancy by an average of eight years.

Cooking also makes the oil and fat in meat go rancid and this increases the number of oxygen radicals and hence of presumptive carcinogens. Protecting ourselves against these large numbers of oxygen radicals should be a most important step in our campaign to avoid cancer. We can do this by increasing our consumption of uncooked food, avoiding burnt or caramelised food and by taking plenty of Vitamin E, Vitamin C, beta-caratene, selenium and uric acid.

COFFEE

One cup of coffee contains 100 milligrams of caffeine which at one time was thought capable of inhibiting DNA repair thereby increasing the likelihood of tumour formation following a mutation. Recently, as a result of a survey of 14,000 coffee drinkers who had been observed for 17 years, coffee has been cleared of this suspicion. Scientists could find no association between coffee and cancer, despite a US survey three years ago that prompted researchers to suggest that it might cause cancer of the pancreas. These findings have been hotly disputed ever since. It is thought that the answer to the relationship between cancer of the pancreas and increased coffee consumption reported by the US scientists has been misinterpreted; it is now suggested that it is the condition itself which may cause the sufferers to drink more of everything, including coffee, due to the body's disturbed glucose tolerance. It is thought that this factor, which would directly affect the amount of coffee consumed, was not taken into account by the US researchers. (*Yudkin et al., Lancet February 1984.*)

On the other hand, it should not be forgotten that browning and burning organic substances such as roasting coffee beans, produces substances which can damage DNA or inhibit its repair faculties. Several such substances have been isolated so it is a good idea to refrain from drinking too many cups of coffee a day. Besides, frequent cups of coffee or tea make people over-tensed and unable to relax properly, thus contributing to stress instead of, as intended, relieving it.

Tea and coffee act both as a drug and a stimulant; as a drug they are habit forming, as a stimulant they are nutritional stressors causing increased general irritability.

Their stimulating effect is due to the caffeine (or theine) they contain. They are refreshing, because they are served hot and because, in our minds, we associate them with comfort and sympathy.

DIETARY FIBRE

Dietary fibre is the medical term for roughage in food; it is the scaffolding that supports plants, giving them their shape and strength. Modern research has shown that as well as preventing constipation it has many other beneficial effects yet it is removed by modern food processing to our great loss. Most fibre is a mixture of substances which passes through our digestive system more or less unchanged and unabsorbed.

It was Dr Denis Burkitt who said that dietary fibre, and in particular bran, might be important in the prevention of bowel cancer. Bran is the husk, or outer shell, of the wheatgrain, and is not used by human digestive enzymes. In whole-wheat there are two types of fibre: crude fibre and dietary fibre (which is finer and about five times as plentiful). It contains complex carbohydrates such as lignin which passes through the bowel totally unchanged, cellulose, hexose and pentose polymers. Pentose polymers are abundant in cereal fibre, present to a lesser extent in other vegetables, but do not occur in potatoes and are thought to produce soft, bulky stools. It is probable that the cancer-reducing effect of fibre is due to the reduced time that the soft bulky stools remain in the bowel. Also, this cancer-reducing effect is increased by altering the total number and proportions of different types of bacteria in the bowel, some of which are capable of destroying carcinogenic metabolites. Furthermore, the presence of phytic acid in bran inhibits the iron-mediated formation of the free oxygen radicals. In this way colonic carcinogenesis can be suppressed by bran and other diets rich in iron-binding phytic acid.

These findings are confirmed by reports from Scandinavia where there is close correlation between bulky stools containing pentose polymer and phytic acid and low large-bowel cancer. This is the case in rural Finland where diets include large amounts of unrefined rye bread; the stools are bulky and the incidence of large-bowel cancer low. The opposite is true in Copenhagen, where the chief difference from the Finnish diet seems to be a much smaller consumption of unrefined cereals.

Because of its vital importance to health, it is worth repeating that eating vegetables, fruit and high-fibre foods, will not only supply far fewer calories, but by virtue of their bulk, will tend to prolong the 'full-up' feeling thus reducing appetite and promoting bowel movement (*intestinal peristalsis*). This is very important because constipation is still one of the commonest disabilities in the affluent West and laxatives are in such great demand that £4 million are spent on them each year in Great Britain and $49 million in the USA.

7·THE THREE VICES: PROMISCUOUS SEX, ALCOHOL AND SMOKING

SEXUAL BEHAVIOUR

Cancer of the neck of the womb seems to be related to the sexual act, since the disease spares nuns and virgins but not nuns who joined their Orders later in life.

It is extremely rare in Jewish women, probably on account of their partners having been circumcised at birth which makes male genital cleanliness easier and reduces the risk of infection. It is uncommon in Parsees, perhaps because their religion is based on purity, which means that they practice meticulous genital hygiene, an invaluable protective measure that is well-worth emulating.

The risk of developing cervical cancer increases with the number of marriages and with the number of extra-marital partners. It is most common in prostitutes. It is also related to the age at which regular sexual intercourse first takes place, the younger the woman, the greater the risk of contracting the disease. The risk is further increased by sexual promiscuity, especially in the 'teens', when the cervix is vulnerable to injury, and is further aggravated by having a venereal infection, particularly if early in life.

There is increasing evidence that the use of barrier contraceptives, sheath or diaphragm (cap), is of great protective value, because the disease is apparently of venereal origin, due to sexually transmitted infection of either the genital *herpes virus II* or one of the many types of *human papilloma virus* responsible for genital warts, which is usually passed from the infected, uncircumcised male during intercourse. Its infectious origin is proved by the fact that the risk of developing the disease depends as much on the number of partners the woman's partner has had, as on the number she has had herself.

The infection tends to occur together in husband and wife and will probably be found to cause the much rarer cancer of the penis. This form of cancer can permanently be prevented by circumcision at birth.

90

The occurrence of genital warts has doubled in frequency in the past eight years, as has the frequency of cancerous lesions of the cervix, especially in young women.

There are two complicating factors:

1. The *herpes simplex II* virus is known to be directly associated with an increased incidence of cancer of the cervix.
2. Smoking has been shown to increase the proneness to the disease in infected cases.

It is thought that cancer of the cervix may arise as a result of the herpes simplex II virus with the human papilloma virus (or, alternatively, nicotine) as the promotor.

The fact that invasive cervical cancer occurs more frequently in oral contraceptive users can be explained on hormonal grounds. The contraceptive hormones increase the reproduction rate of the virus, stimulating the infectious process. That hormones increase the size of genital warts can be seen during pregnancy.

The current frequency of human papilloma virus infection makes two-yearly cervical smears essential, particularly in young women who smoke and are on oral contraceptives.

Cancer of the cervix still kills 4,600 women in the United States and some 2,000 women in Britain each year and more than twice as many under the age of 35 than it did 15 years ago. This may be a reflection on the earlier age at which regular sexual intercourse is started these days in a permissive society where the contraceptive pill, being readily available, encourages this behaviour.

In Iceland where practically all women are screened every 2–3 years the incidence of cervical cancer has dropped by two-thirds, whereas in Norway, where only five per cent are screened it has risen by one-sixth. The UK has a similar programme to that in Norway. At present only the better educated British women seem to attend regularly for screening, yet it is the poorer social classes who, having a much higher incidence of cervical cancer (possibly due to a lower standard of genital hygiene), are at greater risk and who would benefit most by regular screening.

It is estimated that the availability of a regular cervical smear test (called a Pap smear after its originator Dr Papanicolaus) for all young women every two years would reduce the current cervical death rate by half. Even so, more lives would be saved by giving up smoking. The follow-up study of women who refused treatment after abnormalities of the cervix were detected, has proved the great preventive value of the Pap smear.

Summarising, the risk of contracting cervical cancer can therefore be greatly reduced by:

1. Postponing the practice of regular intercourse until well beyond the 'teens'.
2. By using a barrier contraceptive.
3. By having a single partner.
4. By making one's partner, especially if uncircumcised, wash thoroughly behind the foreskin before intercourse.
5. By having a hot bath immediately after intercourse, with scrupulous cleansing of the vagina. This is an additional simple measure of immense protective value.

ALCOHOL

Alcohol has a known carcinogenic effect on organs with which it comes in direct contact such as the tongue, mouth, pharynx and oesophagus. Additionally, since it is broken down in the liver cells, its detrimental effect leads to fatty degeneration of the liver leading first to liver cirrhosis and eventually to liver cancer. Reducing alcohol intake therefore provides a rare opportunity for avoiding cancer at these sites.

The detrimental effect of alcohol and the degree of damage it causes, is directly related to its concentration (beer contains 5 per cent alcohol, wine 10 per cent, sherry 15 per cent and spirits 30 per cent). In America, alcoholic mouth-washes have been found to increase the incidence of mouth-cancer in non-smoking women.

In Britain, alcohol consumption is rapidly getting out of hand and the incidence of liver cirrhosis is up by 50 per cent in the last ten years, while hospital admissions due to alcohol-related diseases are up by 90 per cent in men and 150 per cent in women. In the United States there are 27,700 deaths per year from liver cirrhosis. The permitted daily amount regarded as safe healthwise, is two glasses of wine for women (or one pint of beer) and three glasses of wine for men (or one and a half pints of beer). The American Cancer Society estimate that 3 per cent of all cancer deaths are alcohol-induced. The total figure for 1985 was 472,000.

However, many of the fatal cancers attributed to alcohol can be avoided by not smoking. Even low consumption of alcohol is particularly damaging when associated with cigarette smoking. The two seem to interact, each stimulating the effect of the other, and can often cause cancers of the mouth, pharynx, larynx and oesophagus. These diseases are found more frequently in men employed in alcohol-associated trades such as the French vineyards, the cider-based liqueurs industry in Brittany and Normandy, in publicans and in employees of distilleries and breweries.

Alcohol-induced illnesses, particularly fatty degeneration of the liver leading to fatal liver cirrhosis, affect all social classes, including the executive ranks of business and the professions, especially the medical profession.

The virtue of alcoholic abstinence has received a setback as a result of a piece of misguided advice, in the form of a definite health recommendation. This says that a small amount of alcohol (such as one to two pints of beer, or two to four glasses of wine) taken daily is actually beneficial to health, because it will reduce the risk of a heart attack. It can actually be shown that the increased stickiness of the blood-clot-forming platelets (which tends to pre-dispose to coronary thrombosis) is decreased by small amounts of alcohol. Such increased stickiness occurs as a result of consuming a large fatty meal, which in any case, is never advisable on account of a gain in weight and the increased risk of heart disease. In the absence of large fatty meals, there is no increase in platelet stickiness and therefore, no need for alcohol.

The individual consumption of alcohol in Britain has doubled since it reached its lowest point in 1950, leading to, among other harmful effects, an increase in cancer in men and, though to a lesser extent, in women.

Certain body sites, as already mentioned, are made more susceptible to the development of cancer as a result of an increase in alcohol consumption. The main site is the oesophagus and, although smoking may add to the risk, it has been calculated that regular drinking leads to a 17 times greater incidence of oesophageal cancer in both the USA and France.

As regards oral cancer, heavy drinkers who do not smoke treble their risk of oral cancer and in very heavy drinkers the risk would be even greater. Laryngeal cancer is much more frequent in drinkers than in non-drinkers but this again may be partly due to heavy smoking. The rates of lung cancer and laryngeal cancer in smoking drinkers, however, differ dramatically from those seen in non-drinking smokers; alcohol alone, therefore, may play the more significant role at this particular site.

Liver cancer is much more frequent in alcoholics who had developed cirrhosis first. It is one of the prime functions of the liver to break down alcohol. When an organ as sensitive as the liver is repeatedly bombarded with massive amounts of alcohol, the delicate liver cells first break down in the form of fatty degeneration, which then leads to fibrous scarring; that is cirrhosis. The liver function is lost; as a result the patient can no longer deal with the breakdown of food. He or she will become nauseated, jaundiced and will lose all appetite and energy. The liver tissue, damaged by alcohol, is much more susceptible to malignant change.

The general health of alcoholics suffers because of lack of appetite and the resulting under-nourishment and, since alcohol has no nutritional value, malnutrition. In particular there is vitamin and mineral deficiency, especially of Vitamin B, folic acid, magnesium, iron and zinc.

Whereas liver cirrhosis in alcoholics appears to be a precursor of liver cancer, the increased susceptibility to cancer of the upper digestive and respiratory passages is probably due to direct cellular changes resulting from repeated contact of the tissues with alcohol. This may be most harmful in the oesophagus, where the associated decrease in production of saliva will be most damaging.

It has been suggested that our immunological system functions less efficiently as a result of excessive alcohol consumption and thus leaves us more vulnerable to cancer-causing agents. This attractive and plausible theory still awaits statistical confirmation, but what has been confirmed beyond any doubt is that alcohol exerts its most damaging effect in conjunction with smoking. The chances of a heavy smoker developing oral cancer are 150 per cent greater than those of a non-smoker. But once alcoholic drinks are added, these risks rocket to 1500 per cent. In other words, alcohol enhances the dangerous effects of tobacco and the sites most threatened are the oesophagus and larynx.

Certain geographically-based myths about the special advantages of locally produced drinks are not true. For example, in France it is believed that white wine and the red wine of the south are less damaging, as regards liver cirrhosis, than the red wine of northern France. In Portugal it is said port wine causes cirrhosis but sherry does not. The Germans praise their beer as responsible for the lower incidence of liver cirrhosis. There is no scientific basis to any of these nationalistic claims.

As already stated, the only important determining factor, apart from individual susceptibility, (which, by the way, is greater in women than in men) is the total amount of alcohol consumed, irrespective of the type of drink taken.

Large sums of money have been allocated by the governments of the Western world for an educational campaign to advance public knowledge on the dangers associated with taking drugs. This is important. However, no corresponding campaign is being sponsored in regard to the dangers to life and health from alcohol.

Yet every day £3.5 million are spent on alcohol in Scotland alone.

The annual death toll from drugs in Scotland is 50 deaths, whereas 8,000 die from the over-consumption of alcohol. The corresponding annual figures for the whole of Britain are: 350 deaths from drugs and 60,000 deaths as a result of a national daily spending of £35 million on alcohol.

SMOKING

Every year 100,000 victims, that is one person every five minutes, die unnecessarily from the results of heavy smoking. There is ample, proven evidence of the disastrous effect of cigarettes on health.

The noxious components of tobacco are: tar, nicotine and carbon monoxide. It is the tar in the cigarette which causes lung cancer; it also causes cancer of the mouth, larynx, oesophagus, pancreas and bladder.

Surely every thinking man and woman in the Western world must now be fully aware of the direct link between smoking and lung cancer. The reason why people find it difficult to give it up, once they have started smoking regularly springs from the great physical and emotional dependence on cigarettes produced by the nicotine's pleasurable effects on our senses. Resisting the ever recurring craving for yet another cigarette never ceases throughout one's whole life and represents an ever-present potential threat. This is why it is so important not to start smoking, since weaning oneself off this addiction is so very difficult.

The risks from smoking are influenced by the number of cigarettes and their tar content. Low-tar cigarettes decrease the risk, but smoking two packets of low-tar cigarettes a day carries a higher lung-cancer death rate than one packet of high-tar cigarettes smoked in the same period.

If giving up smoking proves impossible, it is better to smoke not more than six low-tar cigarettes a day, not to inhale deeply and to stub each one out when halfway through. As already seen, the carcinogenic effect of cigarettes is enormously enhanced by alcohol.

The prevalence of smoking in the UK has declined in adult men by one-fifth in the last decade, and is decreasing in women. This is most marked among men in professional and similar occupations, where the proportion of smokers has decreased dramatically. At the other end of the social scale the number of smokers has remained practically constant and more and more youngsters are taking up the habit.

There are now 20 million non-smokers, 10 million ex-smokers and 18 million smokers in the UK. It was as recently as 1976 that for the first time there were more non-smokers than smokers in Britain.

The cost of medical care for the 108,000 people suffering from smoking-related diseases, who have to enter hospital each year, is £111 million. Of these 77,000 will die. Yet children below the age of 16 years spend at least £65 million on cigarettes every year.

A surprisingly quick beneficial effect in health follows the stopping of smoking, particularly in low-tar cigarette smokers, resulting in a substantial reduction in mortality in men under 50 years of age. Cigarette smokers who switch to small cigars run the same risk because most such smokers inhale the cigar smoke; this is not the case in large cigar smokers.

The risk from inhaled cigarette smoke for a 20 cigarette-a-day smoker, apart from the discomfort due to shortness of breath on the slightest exertion and the greater proneness to colds and coughs, is an average life-shortening of about eight years. Those who complain about air pollution from car exhausts and industrialisation should remember that there are 100,000 particles contained in each cubic centimetre of polluted air; by contrast, when smoking we suck in five billion particles per cubic centimetre of smoke directly through the mouth into the lung, without the protective filtering by the nose. Air pollution therefore plays a very minor health threat compared with the risks associated with smoking. Significantly, air in the house of smokers is considerably more polluted than the city air outside. It follows that people who are worried about the effect of air pollution on their lungs should ban smoking in the home as it is a serious occupational hazard.

Non-smoking wives of heavy smokers have a higher risk of developing lung cancer and this risk is the higher the greater the number of cigarettes smoked. What is more, in countries where only a small proportion of women smoke, the effect of passive 'smoking' on lung cancer in women actually becomes more important than that of direct smoking. A 14-year study of 265,000 Japanese men and women concluded that a husband who smoked 20 cigarettes-a-day doubled a non-smoking wife's risk of dying of lung cancer. These findings were confirmed by the American Cancer Society Study in 1981 and by the Louisiana study in 1983.

Estimates of the degree of risk incurred from 'passive smoking' can now be accurately assessed from measurements of urinary cotinine, a metabolite of nicotine, found in the urine of non-smokers breathing other people's smoke.

To conclude: Recent statistics show that 50 per cent of persons still smoking heavily by the age of 35, will be dead by 65; the other 50 per cent will have angina, or high blood pressure, or a stroke, or chronic bronchitis or a leg amputation.

8·HEREDITY AND AGE

HEREDITY AND CANCER
Heredity is a relatively unimportant factor in carcinogenesis. But since growth is controlled by genes and as the two major criteria of cancer are increased rate of reproduction and uncontrolled growth, by implication, genetic factors must play a certain role in all cancers. However, compared with the influence of the environment, the contribution of genetic factors is rather slight for the more common forms of cancer. There is evidence that defects passed in the genes to infants can create a proneness to cancer in later life; in other words, a tendency to a certain type of cancer may sometimes be hereditary and such cancer inheritance is mostly site-specific i.e. the tumour arises in identical organs so that there appears to be a genuine family tendency for bowel, stomach and breast cancer, and to a lesser degree for lung cancer.

BOWEL CANCER
This inherited condition usually develops in existing polyps which mostly line the whole of the large bowel. Without removal of the affected gut, 90 per cent of those affected would die of bowel cancer. *Polyposis coli* is inherited as a dominant trait and the primary cause is an abnormal gene.

STOMACH CANCER
This is more common in the lower social classes, perhaps on account of cigarette smoking and an unhealthy diet. It has a genetic component which is only slight and is greatly influenced by environmental factors. The frequency in near relatives is small: about three per cent of close relatives are likely to develop the disease, as against one-and-a-half per cent in non-related patients. In a study of stomach cancers as many as

97

73 per cent of identical twins were found to be discordant (presence of stomach cancer in only one of the twins). This emphasises the importance of environmental factors. If genetic factors were of greater importance the incidence of cancer in both twins would be much higher.

BREAST CANCER

It is known that childbearing makes a woman less liable to this disease. But breast cancer is less common in childbearing women without a family history of breast cancer than it is in child-bearing women with relatives who have the disease. Therefore a family history of breast cancer in mother, sister, grandmother or aunt is a contributory factor, but it is a relatively unimportant one, when compared with such other predisposing factors as obesity, childlessness, a first menstruation at the age of 10 years, or excessive hard-fat consumption, particularly that of milk-fat (as in butter, cream, cheese and whole milk).

SKIN CANCER

A defect in the production of enzymes that repair DNA damaged by ultraviolet light (the defect having probably been caused by a mutation) is responsible for a rare hereditary skin disease called *Xeroderma pigmentosum*. In this disease oversensitivity to ultraviolet sunlight also produces a tendency to multiple skin cancers on the exposed part of the skin. Pigmentation of the skin is also a hereditary trait that decreases susceptibility to skin cancer by protecting the skin against ultraviolet sunlight.

RETINAL CANCER

Retinoblastoma, a growth affecting the retina, is inherited as a dominant trait; it develops in about one in 18,000 children. About 30 per cent have *unilateral* disease (in one eye only), whilst the remainder have *bilateral* disease (in both eyes).

AGE AND CANCER

It is automatically assumed that cancer, being a degenerative disease, is a natural consequence of growing old and that this is the reason for its prevalence in the elderly. This is wrong because it equates ageing with cancer.

There are two interdependent causes for the high incidence of cancer in old age. The first is a genetic one. As already explained, the probability of any cell suffering a mutation increases in proportion with time, the oddities of life-style and careless attention to diet, smoking, etc. So, the longer we live, the greater the probability will be that even our efficient genetic repair processes will eventually start to break down in one after the other of the controlling genes.

The length of time it will take for such mutations to become established in all the controlling genes will largely depend on the availability of oxygen. Our arteries can be kept young and clear (ensuring a quick, thin bloodstream and thus an excellent oxygen supply for all body tissues) by careful diet and exercise, and mutations have less chance of becoming established when the body cells are oxygen-saturated.

As a direct result of habitual physical inactivity and gluttony, fatty cholesterol-plaques form on the arterial walls, causing, with advancing years, the arteries to harden and the bloodstream to become sluggish and oxygen-depleted. As a result the oxygen-starved cells, which can no longer find enough energy for their continuing healthy survival from blood-oxygen, will try to get this energy from fermenting sugar, a process requiring no oxygen. Normal body cells are *obligate aerobes* (oxygen-requiring cells) and they usually meet their needs by breathing oxygen gas. All cancer cells are *partial anaerobes* (not requiring oxygen for their survival) and their energy needs can be met in great part by fermentation. Although cancer has countless secondary causes, one of these is the replacement of respiratory oxygen gas in normal body cells by fermentation of sugar. This fermentation provides the impetus for carcinogenesis and only occurs when the blood is oxygen-depleted. Therefore, maintenance of an adequate oxygen supply is of great importance at all ages, but particularly so with advancing years.

Clean arteries without fat deposits are achievable only by regular vigorous exercise, because physical activity has dramatic, almost spectacular effects on the body. These are the results of a steadily rising *stroke-volume* (beat) of the heart with regular exercise. The volume of blood pushed out with each heartbeat continues to increase and this has a number of beneficial effects: the bloodstream's speed increases and it gets thinner. By this, oxygenation throughout the body is improved, and there will be no need to meet the cells' energy requirements through fermentation.

During exercise, two substances are released: the prostacyclins and the endorphins. The prostacyclins are *fibrolytic*, which means they prevent the formation of the fatty plaques on the arterial walls. The endorphins promote a sense of well-being and counter depression.

Vigorous exercise also prevents obesity, which is one of the most important contributory causes of cancer.

In short, being lazy is basically being sick and those who do not find time for exercise early on in life will later have to find time for sickness.

9·SCREENING
FOR CANCER

Neither tumour detection at its earliest stage of advancement, nor instant treatment, can guarantee a successful outcome. This worrying uncertainty highlights not only the inadequacy of the treatment methods currently available (with no major improvement in sight), but above all, it shows up cancer's dangerous unpredictability in frequently metastasising while still undetectable. This of course makes a mockery of early screening for cancer at most sites.

Screening programmes have been tried for six anatomical sites: breast, cervix, testes, bladder, melanoma of skin and lung. Only screening for carcinoma of cervix has become established but even this programme leaves a great deal to be desired.

BREAST
In a group of 31,000 women who were screened for breast cancer for three years (with a similar group of women left unchecked) there was a saving of only 38 lives and all of these were older than 50 years; there would therefore seem to be no point in screening women under the age of 50. One of the explanations offered is that in younger women breast cancer may spread too rapidly to be intercepted by screening.

The detection of breast cancer during screening is hailed as a life saved. This is unrealistic and incorrect as much depends on the response to treatment. Post-treatment mortality increases with time after the initial, sometimes apparently successful, treatment. In any event, a woman who has had cancer in one breast has a sixfold chance of developing cancer in the other breast. Unless she tries to change her life-style, the factors which caused the original growth remain unchanged.

The dangers from X-ray mammography used to consist in radiation-induced breast cancer in the organ repeatedly screened. This excess breast cancer incidence becomes apparent some 15 years later. Screening can now provide the best hope of reducing the high breast cancer mortality because modern mammography can now detect a cancer in situ (which is a growth that has not yet developed invasive tendencies), as well as a cancer less than 2cm in diameter (which is vastly superior to clinical examination) and since the X-ray dose with up-to-date apparatus has been reduced from 3 rads to 0.3 rads per exposure. A first or baseline mammographic examination should be carried out between the ages of 35 and 40. Subsequent mammographic examinations should be performed at three-yearly intervals. After the age of 50 annual examinations should be carried out. With the very low doses achieved by modern apparatus and with the use of high speed film or sensitive paper, the potential hazard of inducing breast cancer is negligible.

CANCER OF CERVIX
The frequency of cervical smear tests, when to start these and when to discontinue in old age, varies from country to country. What is similar is the fact that low-risk women get over-screened while the service fails to reach those who need it. In the USA, all sexually active women are screened at three-yearly intervals from their late teens until the age of sixty.

In Britain, probably with an eye to its prohibitive costs, women are first screened when they attend clinics for advice on contraception, pregnancy or venereal disease at the age of 25 years. Other sexually active women usually do not start to have regular cervical smears until the age of 30. Three-yearly screening up to the age of 70 is recommended after this. If practised this could theoretically halve the deaths from cancer of the cervix.

TESTES
Since an *undescended testis* is much more prone to cancer, it is logical to give these boys surgery and bring down the testis from the warmth of the abdominal cavity to the cool scrotal sac. Self-examination of the testes, to detect an uneven area of hardening, should be practised.

BLADDER
Workers in the rubber and dye industries used to be screened regularly for bladder cancer. Every six months a specimen of urine was examined

for malignant cells. Such screening has been found unreliable and has not led to a worthwhile reduction of deaths from bladder cancer.

MELANOMA OF THE SKIN

This tumour which generally arises in a benign mole which had sometimes been present since birth, shows its change to cancer by suddenly starting to grow, to deepen in colour, and/or bleed. Self-examination has been found to increase the success rate in Queensland from a 60 per cent (before the campaign started 15 years ago) to an 88 per cent five-year survival in man and 74 per cent survival in women.

LUNG

No case can be made out for the provision of lung screening as a service, although an annual chest X-ray in the elderly should be routinely carried out. A special case can be made out for selective lung screening within certain industries where smokers are exposed to asbestos, coke, uranium, mustard gas, ether and other chemicals.

SUMMARY

To conclude, routine screening with the exception of cervical cancer, has been proved to be of benefit in certain well-defined high-risk groups, such as retinal cancer in children who have inherited the trait for retinoblastoma, colon cancer in young people with the trait of *polyposis coli*, and skin cancers in persons afflicted with *xeroderma pigmentosum*. The screening service should include a careful follow-up of these genetically handicapped persons.

It would be impracticable to carry out routine screening of people at higher cancer risk for personal reasons, such as smoking, excess-consumption of milk-fat or obesity.

What should be contemplated, in view of the increasing mortality from bowel cancer, is the introduction of routine stool examination which might identify persons at particularly high risk to develop bowel cancer.

A simple home test kit to detect hidden blood in the stool, even before bowel symptoms appear, is now on sale in the USA, and about to be released in the UK. The result of the test, in the form of a change in colour, becomes obvious minutes after spraying the specially prepared paper tissue, to which a sample of the stool has been applied, with the provided detector solution.

This home test has proved as reliable as the routinely used hospital laboratory test for occult blood in the stool.

Since successful surgery for bowel cancer entirely depends on early detection, this simple home test should be mandatory for the overweight meat-eaters and others in the high risk group for bowel cancer.

Whereas a blood test for cancer remains impossible, a number of factors which may contribute to a greater likelihood of contracting cancer can already be estimated in a blood-sample. These include constituents of tobacco, dietary factors, medicines, genetic factors and even DNA damage.

Some information on cancer may however already be gleaned from an ordinary blood test. In all, three substances which may help either to monitor response to treatment in established cases or assist in the detection of a fresh recurrence are readily detectable. They are: *chorionic gonadotrophin* in the rare cancer of the placenta, called *chorio-carcinoma*; the *carcino-embryonic antigen* which is produced by some cancers of the colon and the *alphafetoprotein*, which is found in people with advanced liver cancer. The existence of these substances in the blood has been of great help in the handling of these cases and also in the control of their subsequent disease-free survival.

10·COPING WITH TERMINAL CANCER

PAIN

Pain is usually a late symptom of cancer because an early small growth which does not exert pressure or invade neighbouring structures, is painless. It has no nerves of its own to transmit painful signals to the brain.

It is generally believed that the pain associated with late cancer is too severe to be relievable, but this is not so. Pain can be effectively relieved by morphia, a powerful enough tool for all degrees of pain. Since it can be taken in a watery solution by mouth, a family can manage such medication on its own. Therefore the patient is able to continue leading a near-normal life in the familiar atmosphere of his own home.

Injections of morphia are necessary only for overwhelming pain, which is rare. Otherwise the oral morphia is almost always effective. Instant total pain-relief is a bonus; the maximum good effect usually builds up over a period of two to three weeks. It is important to continue to give morphia to the very end of life because even dying patients need it. Otherwise they develop withdrawal symptoms, which may cause distressing restlessness and even incontinence.

For effective relief of continuous pain, regular four-hourly doses of morphia are necessary throughout 24 hours. This means wakening the patient at night, unless a double dose at bedtime makes this unnecessary.

There are regular side-effects from morphia and these include vomiting, drowsiness, unsteadiness and constipation. The continuation of successful morphia administration depends on the effective control of vomiting (through drugs) and of constipation (through the regular use of laxatives).

Psychological addiction to morphia in cancer patients does not occur, but physical dependence develops after three weeks. Contrary to popular belief, patients do not die more quickly through being on morphia and it should therefore not be regarded as a pre-terminal drug.

Given at the right time, it enables the patient to live a nearly normal life at home for that much longer.

PAIN AND THE EMOTIONS

It is vitally important that all concerned in the care of these patients should understand that the pain they suffer is only in part a purely physical pain. Additionally, there are several psychological components of pain, the more important of these involving emotions like anger, anxiety and depression.

1. Anger: Of course, like that of any other human being, a cancer patient's anger can be a quite normal reaction to an unreasonable delay in making the diagnosis; or it can be caused by the failure of the treatment. On the other hand, anger can be due to less reasonable circumstances, such as the patient's mostly unjustified conviction that he has been abandoned by all his friends. Some feel very bitter at the injustice of being struck down by cancer when others remain healthy.

2. Anxiety: This is a rational feeling of a person who has lost the means of earning an income and who does not know what the future has in store for his or her family. Less justified, but very understandable, is the fear that the pain will become uncontrollable. Of course, in everyone's mind, there is also the fear of death.

3. Depression in a cancer patient is also understandable. After all, the tragic realisation of having personally lost so very much, not only in the way of income, but also in social status and job prestige, produces a depressing feeling of helplessness and hopelessness. This is aggravated even further by the all too frequent presence of uncontrollable insomnia.

From this it will be clear that the relief of cancer pain is not simply a matter of dealing with the purely physical aspect of the pain. There are the other important psychological components that influence how the pain is felt, and these must be taken into consideration when attempting to get rid of it.

The only satisfactory manner of coping with these negative emotions is to sit down with the patient for a series of lengthy talks, during which the many personal points that trouble him must be patiently discussed and explained.

The person looking after a terminal cancer patient has to develop tremendous self-control, so as not to show tears or sorrow. He or she must also display the right mixture of firmness and kindness with which to help the patient gently through his lowest times.

HOSPICES

However desirable it may be for patients to remain in their own homes to the very end, this cannot always happen. Firstly, there are those who live on their own and have no one to look after them and to provide continuous nursing care for an indefinite period. There are families who are too emotional to cope with the stressful situation inevitably surrounding a loved one who is dying of cancer. Towards the end, nursing becomes increasingly heavy, complicated and traumatic. Then there are many cancer patients who do not wish to remain in their homes because they want to spare their nearest and dearest the saddening sight of their death.

How very fortunate therefore that there are such places as cancer hospices. They are a very recent development, especially created for needy cancer patients, so that they can die in comfort, dignity and peace, looked after by a specially trained team of caring, experienced and compassionate nurses. These hospices cope quite beautifully with the many grim problems associated with a progressive, fatal disease, loaded with emotional overtones.

There is still no concensus of opinion with regard to the ideal number of beds in a ward reserved for terminally-ill patients. In the author's opinion there is no doubt whatever that patients should have single rooms which they can regard as their very own, to which they can bring their own furniture, pictures, trinkets and other private possessions, so as to make it a real home-from-home. Yet most new hospices still provide only four-bedded wards, arguing that for patients doomed to die, it may be very reassuring and instructive to witness at first hand the peaceful death of their neighbour in the next bed.

In reality, such deaths in adjoining beds, far from being reassuring, only tend to remind patients that it will be their turn next. Furthermore, most patients, when in the process of dying, are usually screened off by having the curtains drawn around their beds, so their death cannot be observed in any case, which is only as it should be.

Apart from the homely atmosphere that patients are able to create for themselves, single rooms have the advantage of allowing the occupants total freedom. They can choose when to watch television, listen to the radio or settle down for the night. They are able to receive guests at unusual hours and have the luxury of absolute privacy when talking to their visitors. They may talk in confidence without fear of being overheard, and can exchange expressions of tenderness and affection with their loved ones without the risk of being observed.

The decision whether and when to transfer patients to a hospice should be a joint one between the patient, the family, the doctor and the health visitor. Home nursing can sometimes be usefully interrupted by admission to the hospice for a brief period, to allow exhausted relatives a short break from the heavy burden of day and night nursing duties.

The advantages of being looked after in a hospice when suffering from advanced, terminal cancer cannot be measured. What is really striking is the complete transformation of a patient's outlook and attitude, which usually occurs within a very few days of admission. This is due to the very compassionate handling of patients, who soon feel wanted and secure; above all it is the result of the close attention paid to the patient's every need.

It is not surprising that pain and constipation, the two bugbears of home nursing, soon become a thing of the past. Being more relaxed and comfortable, patients soon start needing less and less in the way of pain-relieving drugs and, without strong medication, they become more and more alert and interested in all that is going on around them. Often, surprised visitors cannot believe their eyes to find them so lively and uncomplaining. As a result, visiting becomes a joyful event, instead of a difficult and traumatic experience as patients start to take a renewed interest in their families and their affairs.

In order not to become an impersonal institution, a hospice should be moderately small, resembling a private residence, where everybody knows everybody. Visitors should not have to ring or report to anyone. Visiting hours should be unrestricted, cooking individualised, and the times of serving meals flexible. This would make patients feel more or less at home, because their relatives would have totally free access and could stay as long as they liked.

The happiness of patients at a hospice is in the hands of matron and her nursing staff. Such happiness is directly related to the amount of time set aside by the staff for talking over patients' problems. Patients with cancer, probably more than any other patients, want to be understood and to have matters explained to them. This requires a great deal of time and patience and that is what cancer patients are crying out for.

Some patients may wish to talk about death and they should be allowed to do so, but it is for the patient to take the lead in this matter. No information relating to death should ever be forced on patients. It is unwise and unfeeling to hazard a guess at life-expectancy, even when asked to do so, because the exact length of the final stages of cancer is unpredictable.

Relatives should also be involved in these discussions, and they must be prepared for the patient's eventual death. Although such loss will always be very sad, it is made far more bearable when it is faced squarely and in advance.

To conclude, pre-terminal patients feel safest at home with their families and home will always be the best place to die. However, if this is not possible, a hospice provides an admirable alternative since it allows the patient to die peacefully and in pleasant surroundings.

Any decision regarding admission to the hospice for however long must not be made without the patient's consent, provided, of course, he is still sufficiently alert to be able to make rational decisions. In fact, provided this is the situation, the patient's opinion in this respect is the most important of all.

A new idea, prompted by the need for further extension and improvement of terminal cancer care at home, is the Community Health Team. This consists of a terminal care doctor, a secretary, a number of nurses and a social worker. The team is available to advise on all problems concerning the care of cancer patients in their homes right up to, and even beyond, the patient's death. Usually the team is represented at the patient's funeral, and post-bereavement counselling is provided as a matter of course. It is in the interest of patients and their families to notify the team early on so that there is ample time for its members to get to know their individual situation. This will allow the team to be of more help when it becomes necessary.

UNORTHODOX TREATMENT

Many patients with incurable cancer, when told by their doctors that further treatment would be pointless, may refuse to accept the finality of this chilling verdict. Instead they start searching for someone prepared to continue with any form of treatment in the forlorn hope that success may be possible after all.

Their situation may be heartlessly exploited by deceitful charlatans who only too readily assure the patient that their own simple form of treatment is bound to succeed. This promise will only cause further heartache as soon as the patient realises, as he surely will, that treatment has failed.

Sometimes patients, anxious to avoid all unpleasant side-effects of treatment, may decide to choose the simple method offered by the charlatan, in preference to one of the three old-established and proven methods for cancer, namely surgery, radiotherapy and chemotherapy. This ill-advised decision may well cost some patients their lives.

What makes quack methods so attractive for patients and their worried relatives is the offer of an almost perfect-sounding, very simple treatment, totally free of unpleasant side-effects, which usually promises to result in a lasting cure. To make these assurances is unethical and no qualified doctor would be prepared to raise a patient's hopes in the knowledge that they are likely to be dashed before long.

But charlatans are a special group of people, mostly very charming and persuasive. They share certain characteristics: first and foremost they have only one type of treatment which they are content to use for all forms of cancer; then they diagnose a condition as cancer when, in fact, it is not malignant (they never bother to carry out a biopsy to confirm their diagnosis). To make their diagnosis they use very personal methods. These are different from the established procedures and quite unacceptable as proof of a diagnosis by any properly qualified doctor.

The results of their usually secret form of treatment are not published in scientific journals; instead they rely for publicity on personal testimonials of patients who have supposedly been cured in the past. But many of these cured patients only *thought* that they had cancer, had not consulted an orthodox practitioner, and went along to be reassured. Instead they were instantly offered treatment which they were too surprised to refuse and so were cured of a disease they never had!

Perhaps the success of a cancer charlatan lies to some degree in the fact that the qualified cancer specialist has a clinical and too scientific approach. The specialist, who should *always* offer his patient strong emotional support and hope, sometimes fails to do so. The charlatan knows that his success depends on filling this need, and exploits it to the full.

The most common currently popular quack remedies are Laetrile (a compound made of apricot kernels), which is also called Amygdal or Vitamin B17 (although it is not a vitamin), the so-called mega-vitamin therapy, where massive doses of vitamins are prescribed without any scientific justification, coffee enemas and other so-called 'cleansing' enemas, which are all equally scientifically unsound, hypnotherapy, acupuncture, iridology and faith healing, including the laying on of hands. We know of no scientifically acceptable evidence of miracle cures for cancer brought about by any one of these unorthodox methods.

The standard conventional therapy should *always* come first. If need be it can be given simultaneously with an unconventional treatment. If however a quack method alone is taken first, it can cost the patient's life, because when these methods eventually prove unsuccessful and, months later, the hapless patient returns very sick for further help, it may be too late and orthodox doctors will have no treatment to offer.

When all orthodox treatment has failed and the disconsolate patient explicitly asks to see an unqualified practitioner, this request should not be turned down, because the hope which is engendered in the patient's mind, by receiving further therapy, may make him feel better for a time. Only in such circumstances is unorthodox treatment justifiable. In all other circumstances cancer charlatanery must be considered a deceitful use of unproven methods to treat cancer, practised purely for financial gain.

11·MIND OVER MATTER

STRESS AND EMOTIONS

Stress has a debilitating effect on the body's immune system. Though it is not the actual cause of illness, in a borderline condition it may be the determinant factor which swings the balance.

Stress is a harassed feeling which is experienced when our mind's integrity is challenged by a stressor, usually an intensely disturbing emotion or an unsuccessful struggle.

Stress is neither good nor bad, it is simply a fact of life. What is important is the way we react to it. For some it is the spice of life and they respond with alertness and positive action. Others respond with distress. This passive response leaves some irreversible mental scars and has a suppressive effect on the immune system, making the individual more prone to psychosomatic disease which is a real physical illness due to the body's reaction to its own stressed and troubled mind.

It is not unusual that the onset of illnesses such as cancer can be related to an upset emotional state. For example, in a study of cancer in identical twins, the twin with cancer had recently been through an emotional upheaval, whereas the other twin's life had been tranquil. The existence of such a psychosomatic link has been known since 537 BC, when the respected Greek physician Galen first noted that melancholy and depressed women were more apt to develop breast cancer than cheerful ones.

Today's consumer society is intensely competitive. People are often in a state of constant nervous strain and tension and so are particularly prone to stress-related psychosomatic sickness.

Some illnesses seem more subject to emotional influences than others but evidence is building up to suggest that emotions play an important part in virtually all diseases from the common cold to cancer. There was a time when the common cold was thought to be transmitted directly by exposure to germs. Now it can be shown that we catch a cold when our immune system is weakened and stress has a potent weakening effect on the immune system. Similarly stress, badly handled, plays a part in who gets cancer.

Hope and optimism, on the patient's part, can work wonders because the patient's imagination, when unafraid, is a most powerful ally. By contrast, when weighed down by anxiety, a frightened mind represents a serious threat to health, as a result of its damaging effect on the immune system. Anything that affects our immune system has the potential to aid many disease processes, including cancer. In the study of three sets of twins with leukaemia, the twin who developed the disease was always the twin who had experienced a psychological upheaval right before the onset of the disease; the other twin had not. It looks as if sometimes a psychological trauma might be the prime factor in cancer, even stronger than physical weakness. Other studies have confirmed this link between the onset of signs of cancer and an emotional upheaval such as adultery, separation, loss, redundancy and bereavement. Some workers suggest that it is our reaction, the way we handle and respond to stress, that is the key to whether or not we develop cancer. It is said that it is usually the quiet, non-aggressive, acquiescent person who is found more susceptible to contracting cancer, the so-called cancer-prone personality who tends to bottle up all feelings, including anxieties and worries.

But any theory which says that diseases are caused by mental states and can be cured by will-power, should always be viewed with suspicion, because we do not fully understand the nature of disease. Moreover, there is a modern tendency for psychological explanations to be enlisted as causes for a variety of diseases.

However, in one form of cancer, namely breast cancer, the casual link between mental distress and the disease is not purely hypothetical. The development of breast cancer is greatly feared by many women. There is, therefore, a real danger in this instance, that some women might so mismanage their emotions as actually to contribute to its very development. If they can react to it in a positive way they will begin to be less afraid but nevertheless they will need constant support and encouragement for many months. Feelings of anxiety can do harm only as long as they are bottled up. Once they are brought out into the open and discussed, they lose much of their terror and become defused; merely voicing one's feelings freely avoids the build-up of nervous tension.

Additionally, prayer and contemplation may help to acquire a more relaxed attitude of mind. Meditation (on the other hand) is still considered scientifically unproven in its effect, and there are few reputable centres where this ancient method of mental relaxation is accepted as orthodox treatment. Relaxation techniques, like meditation, which involve repeating a phrase or a prayer in comfortable quiet surroundings, have been in use throughout the world for thousands of years and their beneficial effect is unquestionable. This technique of 'mindless' prayer is thought to reduce the excessive amounts of the hormone *noradrenaline*, which is produced under stress.

A certain kind of quiet disposition is necessary to acquire the art of meditation. Just as some people lack an eye for colour or an ear for music, so it is with many who try to learn to meditate. They find it difficult to relax sufficiently to be able to eliminate their surroundings and their own active thoughts from their mind. This is a necessary prerequisite which then will allow their consciousness to lapse into a dreamy state where all is calm, quiet and peaceful. It is this state of tranquility which will generate the inner harmony which is so invigorating for the mind because of the associated reassuring feeling that all is serene and beautiful.

In man, stress has a damaging effect on the immune system. When the emotional upheaval is short-lived it leaves the body vulnerable for short periods of time. If, however, the stressful state continues for long, the body may be left defenceless.

EXERCISE

Even more tangible evidence of the interaction between mind and body was discovered in the mid-1970s by the identification of the body's own morphia-like substances, called endorphins, which are capable of relieving pain and anguish, as if they were opiates. Regular exercise is known to produce high levels of these endorphins and those who exercise regularly are capable of producing endorphins not only in greater amounts but also more quickly in stressful situations. This means that active people may handle everyday tensions better than inactive types. Our well-being and long-term health is therefore dependent to a certain extent on how determined we manage to be. Regular exercise, by producing high levels of endorphins relieves stress, strain and most types of depression. This is a much better way of relieving the cycle of built-up tensions than employing, as is customary these days, the caffeine of coffee, which only masks rather than relieves these tensions.

If it is to do us any good, exercise should be taken regularly for a period of not less than ten minutes, at least every other day – throughout our entire lifetime. A person who does nothing for a month loses 80 per cent of his or her physical condition and thereby considerably weakens the body's immune defence capability. The more obvious advantage of regular exercise is a healthier heart. Another invaluable bonus of an exercised body is that it provides a much better home for that intangible thing called our soul and in so doing strengthens our immune defences against all kinds of illnesses including cancer.

Another advantage is the absence of flab, because no fat accumulates in a physically active body. Excess fat is almost always due to a little too much rest as well as a little too much food! Physical activity and nutrition are closely related. People who exercise and eat moderately usually stay slim.

It should always be remembered that even in extended vigorous exercises, little of the massive energy contained in dietary fat and sugar is used up; that is why there are so many unsuccessful overweight joggers who, unless they cut down on fats, sugar and alcohol, will always remain fat.

What all too few of us realise is that at a time of personal tragedy or when there is a set-back to our hopes or expectations, vigorous exercise can be remarkably effective in raising our flagging morale, thereby also protecting our threatened immunological defence system from being weakened by our low spirits.

Actually the first step to physical fitness is a mental one: it is one of motivation. Once the mind is made up to exercise regularly, the rest will be less difficult, but we must not be over-ambitious. The intensity and duration of the exercise must be adapted to one's age and general condition. The main objective of fitness is to remain fit enough to continue having fun. In addition, due to the increased pumping capacity of the heart, our quality of life will improve and we will not age prematurely.

There is conclusive evidence that people fortunate enough to be able to engage in regular sporting activities are, as a result of the healthy exercise, usually in excellent mental and physical condition. They are generally relaxed and sleep well; they worry less and they have no desire to over-eat or smoke, nor do they crave alcohol. Not only is their blood pressure normal, their pulse rate is slow at rest, and even more important, it increases only slightly on exertion.

Outdoor sports afford the added bonus of natural unfiltered sunlight, which is essential for good condition. Natural light affects the body's hormone system after entering the eyes through the pupils. This results in a general sense of well-being and lessens tiredness. This explains why natural sunlight has such a very significant association with a person's mood. It doesn't matter how exercise is taken; whether in the form of the 'daily dozen' or taking a long, brisk walk instead of driving the car or taking a bus; running upstairs two at a time rather than taking the lift; cycling long distances or energetically digging the garden.

12·FUTURE CANCER RESEARCH

Thanks to earnest and painstaking research into its many aspects much progress has been made in our understanding of cancer. However, the chances that any of the discoveries being made will be turned into improved survival rates remain small.

Two examples will be enough to explain why this should be so, by illustrating how each new discovery creates a whole string of fresh problems, which need solving first.

1. A certain substance in our body called an oncogene, produced as part of the healing process when we injure ourselves, has been found to promote the growth of certain cancer cells, including those in the bones and other connective tissues. A similar oncogene can be formed by fragments of genetic material known to be associated with viruses which cause cancer in animals. If this substance were to be produced in large amounts in the absence of injury, it could lead to uncontrolled cell growth, typical of cancer. There may well be other oncogenes which are concerned with the control, rather than the promotion of cancerous growth but are yet to be found.

2. The second fresh discovery concerns the effects of a virus causing leukaemia in chickens and also malignant change in human skin cells. This leukaemia virus has a gene which, although it originates in chickens, also exists in human beings. The gene produces a substance (a protein) which controls the growth of skin cells. However, the copy of this gene, carried by the chicken virus, is defective and this defective gene, when introduced into normal cells, induces them to become cancerous.

Once the nature of the chemical process, at the point where the cancer virus intervenes, is determined, a search for potential new drugs, which would interfere with this reaction, can start. Many chemicals will have to be tested before the right drug is found and that will take a long, long time.

13·CONCLUSIONS

Of all the words in a doctor's vocabulary none is as feared as the word *cancer*. It is this fear that makes people so nervous and gullible about the disease.

As a result, any cancer claim, even when wholly unsubstantiated, is all too readily believed, particularly when repeated often in the media. Into this category falls the alleged cancer threat from chemical food-additives such as preservatives, colourants, flavourings, fertilisers, herbicides, insecticides and pesticides. There are, in fact, 314 listed additives under the UK Food Act of 1984. They are the only ones that have been tested and officially passed as safe in Britain. Additionally, there are some 3,000 flavourings which, although untested, are equally safe for those of us who react normally.

In people with known allergic reactions such as asthma, eczema, urticaria, hay fever, headaches and childhood hyper-activity etc., a few additives have been known to provoke some of these allergic reactions. But, if so predisposed, these reactions can also be caused by such simple foods as milk, cheese, eggs, wheat, strawberries, prawns, oysters and, in some people, even by taking aspirin. What is rarely realised that even stress, due to unresolved emotional or other problems, can produce the above reactions. When people prone to allergic reactions develop fresh allergic reactions, they should always bear in mind the possibility of these being due to an additive and should choose new foods with care.

Using a simple analogy of colour-blindness, we find that just as those of us who are colour-blind should not become engine drivers, because this would be somewhat hazardous, so it is risky for an allergic person to indulge indiscriminately in all kinds of new foods. This should, however, not stop the rest of us from becoming engine drivers, or from enjoying with impunity foods containing all kinds of additives.

It is the consensus of informed medical opinion that food additives make no contribution to any single serious illness, including cancer, and the suggestion that some additives are linked with cancer and other serious illnesses are simply untrue. Despite their extensive use during the last 30 years, no cancer deaths had been caused by them during this period.

The presence of additives in our food can, therefore, be disregarded by all those not prone to allergic reactions, which is just as well, because practically all food lines contain additives and it is virtually impossible, and totally unnecessary nowadays, to avoid them.

Large sections of the population still remain sceptical and incur a great deal of unnecessary expense in their efforts to avoid all foods containing these. It would be far more profitable healthwise for the public to concentrate on stopping some of today's habitual dietary excesses because of the direct link which exists between opulence, overweight and that special group of diseases, so aptly named 'cancers of affluence'. There is convincing evidence that in our industrialised and over-fed third of the world, 'having it too good' is one of the prime contributory factors responsible for the high incidence of such cancers of affluence as cancer of the large bowel, rectum, gall bladder, breast, prostate, uterus, ovary and possibly pancreas.

What is more, over-eating when indulged in regularly every day over 20 or more years will inevitably substantially increase the likelihood of contracting not only one of the cancers of affluence, but also one or the other of the more disabling degenerative diseases, such as heart disease, high blood pressure, a stroke or diabetes.

We also know now that consumption of hard fats, that is those of animal origin such as milk-fat (contained in whole milk, butter, cheese and cream), as well as of the fat in red meat, is associated with a higher frequency of breast cancer. It is suggested that this association may be limited to pre-menopausal women, in whom that risk may be quite substantial.

What is more, this high breast-cancer rate could be further reduced by reversing the current trend towards an early menarche (first menstruation), which is associated with reaching the weight of 7st 2lb (46 kg) at the age of 10½ years, instead of 17.

On the credit side, it has been shown that there is a lower cancer rate in ethnic population groups who, by virtue of religion, ancient custom and beliefs or simply by force of reduced circumstance, have led a restrained, frugal life of austerity devoid of all forms of dietary excess, a conclusion so convincingly documented by the British nation's vastly improved post-war health, resulting from the nutritional constraints of wartime rationing.

Although we live in enlightened times, these important epidemiological findings are not generally known. In fact, it is estimated that of the people currently living in the Western world, only about 33 per cent are living in anything approaching the right way. The remaining 67 per cent seem totally unaware that there is an element of self-destruction, not only, as already stated in regular overeating, but also in regular over-consumption of alcohol and in heavy smoking.

There is also an element of self-destruction in sexual promiscuity at any age, but especially so in the teens, and in prolonged physical inactivity, particularly as we advance in age, from 40 years onwards. Last but not least, and probably very surprisingly to many, there is a grave element of self-destruction in the insatiable materialistic greed of today's Western consumer society. It is the constant preoccupation and the ever-present hunger for more and better material possessions which creates a permanent state of increased strain and mental tension and this in turn causes a greater proneness to psychosomatic illness, which is not a hysterical condition requiring psychological attention, but a real, stress-induced physical illness, brought on by the body's reaction to its own stressed and troubled mind.

The solution to these many self-inflicted problems will come within our grasp once we shall have decided that staying healthy is what we want most of all in life, because only then shall we find the motivating willpower necessary to make us adhere to the principles enunciated in the 10 health lessons below.

10 HEALTH LESSONS

The chances of avoiding cancer and premature ageing as well as many of today's disabilities caused by degenerative diseases are immeasurably enhanced by constant observance of 10 health-precepts summed up in the two five-letter acronyms: 'FACTS' and 'SMART'.

The acronym 'FACTS' stands for Fat, Alcohol, Cigarettes, Tension and Sugar: for long-term good health all five are best avoided, if at all possible.

The acronym 'SMART' stands for Serenity, Moderation, Activity, Roughage and Trying. Early adoption of all five is of paramount importance, because each one in turn complements the beneficial effects of the others in the quest for lasting health and fulfilment.

Serenity: A high quality of life depends as much on a relaxed mind and a deep faith, as on physical well-being.

Moderation: This quite indispensable prerequisite for long-term health can be successfully sustained only if based on self-discipline, willpower and motivation.

Activity: Without regular physical exercise the clean arteries necessary for a free-flowing, oxygen-rich bloodstream which provides the vital supply of nutrients and oxygen to the tissues will be impeded, leaving the cells malnourished and unpurified, that is, laden with waste products which cannot be cleared.

Roughage: Crude, fibre-containing foods are easily the most important constituent of one's diet since they absorb toxic substances from the bowel and expedite their elimination by increasing the peristaltic movement of the gut.

Trying: It is only by constant trying that the control and conquest of one's habitual weaknesses will become second nature.

GLOSSARY

Alimentary – pertaining to the absorption of nourishment

Anaemia – reduction in the number of the red cells or in the content of haemoglobin, or both

Antibody – protein substance which neutralises a corresponding antigen

Aorta – the large artery arising from the heart and supplying blood to the whole body

Barium enema – a contrast medium used to outline the bowel

Basal layer – skin layer underlying the dermis

Benign – non-malignant, not cancerous

Benzpyrene – carcinogenic compound composed of hydrogen and carbon

Biopsy – examination of a piece of tissue from a living body under a microscope

Blast cells – immature white cells which arise in the bone marrow, being forerunners of leucocytes

Bronchi (bronchoscopy) – the air tubes leading from the windpipe into the lungs which allow passage of a lighted telescope for examination of their appearance

Calcification – a deposit of lime in any tissue in the form of a dense deposit of calcium

Carcinogenesis – the process of production of malignant cells

Carcinogens – substances which produce malignant change in a cell leading to development of cancer

Carcinoma – cancer arising in epithelial sheets covering the body surface or organs and linings of internal structures.

CAT – is short for computed axial tomography. An ingenious X-ray apparatus which rotates around the recumbent patient to produce salami-thin transverse body or brain slices, which allow early detection of abnormalities, in particular space-occupying lesions such as a brain tumour or brain haemorrhage in the head, or enlarged lymph nodes or cancer in the body

Catecholamines – a group of compounds that have the effect of stimulating the sympathetic nervous system, such as adrenalin

Catheter – is a hollow tube used for passage of fluids usually from the bladder

Cauterise – to burn by means of applying a heated metal to living tissue, usually to destroy or arrest haemorrhage

Cervix – neck of the womb

Chemotherapy – use of drugs to treat cancer and infections

Cholesterol – a fatty substance originating in animal tissues

Colostomy – operation to make artificial opening for the colon in the anterior wall of the abdomen

Contact inhibition – arrest of tissue growth on coming into contact with adjoining tissue of a different kind

Decalcify (recalcify) – loss, i.e, removal of calcium (its deposition)

Dermis – the skin layer which lies beneath the epidermis

Detoxify – to remove or to neutralise toxic substance

Duodenum – the first ten inches of the small intestine, beginning at the lower end of the stomach

Dysplasia – defective growth of a tissue

Epileptiform – resembling an epileptic seizure

Endocrine – internal secretion of the ductless glands

Enzyme – protein which acts as catalyst

Epidemiological – resulting from study of nature and distribution of diseases worldwide

Epidermis – superficial part of skin overlying dermis

Epithelium (epithelial) – sheet of cells making up skin or other covering membranes or lining of tubes

Familial – affecting several members of one's family

Gene – part of chromosome transmitting hereditary characters

Genetic code – blueprint for identical cell reproduction

Haemoglobin – the colouring matter of the red corpuscles

Hydrolyse – breaking down of substance with addition of water

Immunological – appertaining to resistance to infection due to presence of antibodies

Inducer – substance facilitating a reaction
Initiator – substance initiating cellular chain reaction which may lead to cancer
Integral dose – cumulative dose
Intracranial – inside the skull
Intrinsic – inherent, peculiar to a part

Lactation – the period of suckling
Lesion – morbid change in the function or structure of an organ
Lymph nodes – glands making up lymph chain
Lymphatic – belonging to the system of lymph nodes
Lymphoblastic leukaemia – cancer of the bone marrow, made up of immature cells called lymphoblasts
Lymphosarcoma – a type of cancer arising in the lymphatic system

Malignant – virulent, possibly fatal, the opposite to benign
Membrane – a thin layer of tissue
Metabolism (metabolites) – the changes taking place in living tissues
Metastases – secondary or satellite growths appearing at a distance from the original cancer
Mutagen – substance capable of inducing cancer
Mutation – intracellular change in genetic code leading to malignancy

Neurological – appertaining to diseases of the nervous system

Oestrogen – hormone secreted by ovaries
Organic – relating to living matter
Oxidant – a substance with free oxygen producing oxides on chemical combination
Oxidation – chemical combination with oxygen
Oxygenation – saturation with oxygen

Palliative – designed to relieve only, not to cure
Pancreas – sweetbread. A gland situated behind duodenum
Pharynx – space connecting mouth to oesophagus
Pituitary gland – endocrine gland at base of skull
Platelet – blood cell concerned with clotting
Plasma – liquid in which blood cells are suspended
Polycyclic hydrocarbons – substances formed of hydrogen and carbon
Polyps – a small simple benign tumour
Proctosigmoidoscope – viewing of the rectum and lower part of large

bowel (colon) with a periscope-like instrument introduced via anus

Prognosis – outlook on future, opinion on probable course of disease

Promoter – a substance or circumstance enhancing a biological reaction

Prostate – a male gland situated at the base of the bladder

Prosthesis – replacement of absent organ or limb

Protein – compound made up of many amino-acids

Radio-mimetic – resembling effect produced by radiation

Radiotherapy – treatment by ionising radiation

Retina – delicate net-like membrane covering the eye back-ground

Rectum – terminal part of large bowel

Regression – reverting to a smaller size

Resection – a surgical removal

Sarcoma – a malignant tumour composed of bone, muscle or connective tissue cells

Secretion – the active production of a liquid by cells

Selenium – a naturally occurring mineral

Stoma – an artificial opening

Stroma – connective tissue base

Structuring – the manner in which a tissue is organically formed

Suture – a stitched up wound

Terminal (pre-terminal) – nearing death

Ultrasound – an apparatus using the echo of soundwaves to determine the size and nature of deep-seated structures

Undescended testes – a testicle which has remained inside the abdomen

Uterus – womb

Vulva – the external female genital organ

INDEX

ACKNOWLEDGEMENTS

This book could not have been written without using material appearing in other publications on cancer and the author wishes to thank all those who supplied such information in their works and so helped with researches for this book.

Particular thanks are due to:

Michael Alderson, *The Management of Malignant Disease Series, The Prevention of Cancer, 1982, Edward Arnold*
Denis Burkitt, *Don't Forget Fibre in Your Diet, 1983, M. Dunitz*
John Cairns, *Cancer Science and Society, 1978, W. H. Freeman & Co.*
R. Doll and R. Peto, *The Causes of Cancer, 1981, Oxford University Press*
A. E. H. Emery, *Elements of Medical Genetic, 1971, Churchill Livingstone*
Laurence Morehouse and Leonard Gross, *Total Fitness in 30 Minutes a Week, 1972, Granada Publishing Ltd*
Miriam Polunin, *The Right Way to Eat, 1980, Granada Publishing Ltd*
Susan Sontag, *Illness as Metaphor, 1978, Penguin Books*
Basil A. Stoll, *Mind and Cancer Prognosis, John Wiley & Sons*
Otto Warburg, *The Prime Cause and Prevention of Cancer, 1969, Engl. Ed. by Dean Burke Konrad Triltsch, Wurzburg, Germany*
Elizabeth Whelan, *Preventing Cancer, 1980, Sphere Books Ltd*
Robert Twycross and Sylvia Lack, *Oral Morphine in Advanced Cancer, 1984, Beaconsfield Publishers Ltd*
O. Carl Simonton, Stephanie Matthews-Simonton, James L. Creighton, *Getting Well Again, 1978, Bantam Books*
Patrick Holford, *Vitamin Vitality, 1985, William Collins Sons & Co. Ltd*
Arnold E. Bender, *Health or Hoax, 1985, Elvendon Press*
Harold Glucksberg, Jack W. Singer et al, *Cancer Care, 1980. The John Hopkins University Press.*
M. P. Vessey and Muir Gray, *Cancer: Risks and Prevention, 1985, Oxford University Press*

The author wishes to express his great indebtedness to Mrs Carol Robinson for her invaluable assistance with the numerous researches and for her admirable forbearance in coping with countless amendments to the typescript.